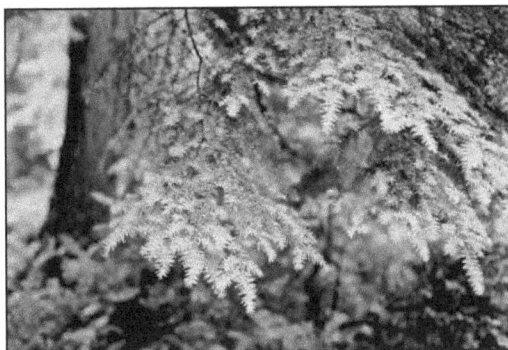

The Tree Is Medicine

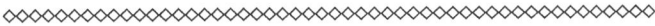

◇◇◇

Infant Mortality at Cedar Bay

Barbara Mould Young, MN, MHP, RN

Pisces Publications
409 Thomas St. SW
Olympia, WA 98502

ISBN 978-0-9894430-9-8

While based on actual events, names and details have been changed.

Photography by Katherine Flenniken unless otherwise indicated.
Back cover photo of author by Charlie Keck

Design by Fletcher Ward

Set in Agaramond Pro 8/19

Dedicated to

The Women of the Circle

and

The Indian Leader, Madzu

Table of Contents

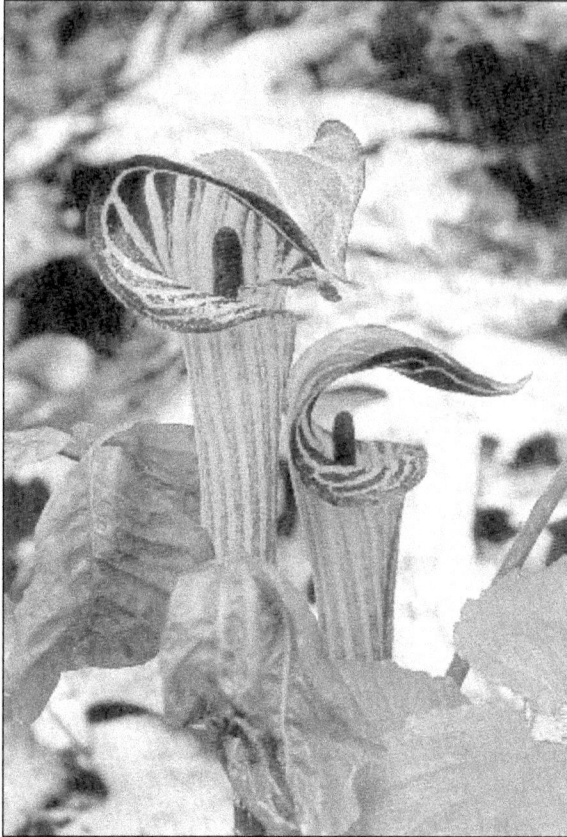

Post card from the Ohio Historical Society
—Photographer unknown

My mother loved the jack-in-the-pulpit and always pointed it out to me on hikes in an Ohio forest. It is a true sign of spring and signifies re-birth after a hard winter. It is confirmation of the circle of life.

Preface

The flagger woman, in her bright orange safety vest with neon yellow stripes, commands me to stop. Traffic from the opposite direction passes over the one piece of road intact after the recent ice storm. A giant backhoe, just over the embankment, moves tons of small rocks to shore up the fallen road. The forest is clear-cut in all directions. There is not enough vegetation to hold water from the storm. Mudslides collapsed the roadbed. Waiting for clearance, I think of trees and their relationship to our lives. I remember Ohio.

◆ ◆ ◆ ◆ ◆

The tree merit badge in Mrs. Gallagher's Girl Scout Troop 535 at E.J. Brown School in Dayton was my favorite badge. I collected and pressed leaves from fifteen trees, including sugar maple, red maple, silver maple, white and red oaks, chestnut oak, poplar, and ginkgo. Pointed leaves, rounded leaves, leaves with symmetrical and asymmetrical veins.

I grew up with two of the most radiant sugar maples on Fernwood Avenue. Fernwood was a blaze of red, yellow and orange in the fall. In summer, I sat on the curb in front of my house under a leaf canopy and felt the warm rainwater flowing over my feet. In the backyard a mighty oak tree cradled my brother's tree house. One time we hauled up a pot of green beans to string and snap, preferring to sit, talk, and work in the tree house instead of a hot kitchen. The other large tree in the backyard was a black walnut. My rope swing hung from its tall branches. Two glorious maples took up the entire front yard—leaving no room for grass on either side of the front walk.

Trees. My mother, who studied speech at Miami University in the early 1920s, would recite poems to project her voice, quell her loneliness, and sustain her confidence. One of her favorite poems was by Joyce Kilmer, a World War I front line artillery man. I memorized it just by hearing it recited so frequently.

Trees

Joyce Kilmer

I think that I shall never see
A poem lovely as a tree.

A tree whose hungry mouth is prest
Against the earth's sweet flowing breast;

A tree that looks at God all day,
And lifts her leafy arms to pray;

A tree that may in Summer wear
A nest of robins in her hair;

Upon whose bosom snow has lain;
Who intimately lives with rain.

Poems are made by fools like me,
But only God can make a tree.

◆ ◆ ◆ ◆ ◆

Now, the colorful deciduous trees of my youth are replaced in the Pacific Northwest with Sitka spruce, Douglas-fir, western hemlock and western red cedar. The rich smell of evergreens on hikes into Olympic National Park and the Cascade Mountains provides solace and relief from city life. Opportunities for these forest hikes diminish as more and more logs are carted to pulp mills to satisfy our unquenchable thirst for paper.

The flagger turns her stop sign to SLOW, my signal to proceed. The nose of an empty logging truck behind me nudges me out of my reverie. The light snow and cold temperature remind me to beware of black ice. If I am not careful, I could go over the bank.

◆ ◆ ◆ ◆ ◆

The chairman of the tribe is Thomas Greyhawk. He asked me to take the position of program manager for the grant-funded investigation into the high rate of infant mortality in his tribe. He made this request in spite of my culture's history with his tribe, in spite of my previous work with the unresponsive state bureaucracy, in spite of my training exclusively in western healing arts, in spite of the color of my skin. Perhaps he hopes that my connection with the state department of health and my willingness to write detailed reports will generate more useful contacts and additional funds for preventive health programs.

The tribe is on the brink of extinction. They are losing babies. They are losing elders. Without hope for the future and without the wisdom of their elders, they are grieving. They mourn the loss of culture, of land, of their dance and language, even of their traditional food. They want to hope. They want a return to health. They want to prevent further deaths and ensure healthy pregnancies. New births could return hope for their future. They want healthy elders who can recall and teach the traditional ways. They seek their own health care system in order to be self-reliant. They seek economic independence. They wish to actively design and implement a path to a healthy future.

It was early in fall when I came into this community. I am a nurse, trained in a prominent school of nursing with advanced degrees—which means little in Indian Country. Many of those in the white healthcare community thought that I was brought to this place only to solve the mystery of a high infant mortality rate on the reservation. Perhaps some tribal members thought that I was brought here to provide access to western-style medical care. Only the Great Spirit understands the true purpose of the work, solves the mysteries that perplex us all, and directs us on the path to health. It is for us to listen, to learn, and to believe that communication can support our co-existence in this region and in the global community. This is a story of shared healing.

In the following pages, I share ancient wisdom of the medicine wheel as I have come to understand it. I share the lessons from this tiny village, with their practice of connected community. As I travel further from my state office cubicle and deeper into the forest and canoe culture, I learn more about myself, my own heritage and culture.

What *were* the causes of infant mortality? Was it a toxic environment? Was it a lack of access to health care? Was it a lack of industry, jobs, adequate income? Was it poverty? Was it alcoholism, diabetes, hepatitis, heart disease or cancer? Was it nutrition and moving away from a traditional diet? Was it loss of land, language, song, dance, and ceremony? Was it spirit loss or soul sickness? There were few remaining elders of advanced age. In a culture where the health and wellness of the elders and children is a good indicator of the health of the community, the tribe was out of balance.

The stories in these pages are of a small Indian nation whose ancestors inhabited the coast, rivers, and forests of the Pacific Northwest, and more specifically, a limited tract of land on a bay that empties into the Pacific Ocean, a short distance north of the confluence of the Columbia River. Clues to the answers were hidden from easy access; they were embedded, waiting to be discovered. This small tribe, descendants of the Canoe People, can help us study the currents, chart the trip, and keep the keel on course.

I share these stories in order to increase cultural awareness and to make connections between peoples of diverse cultures. This is a story of a tribe in mourning for its lost infants, a tribe that is uncertain of its future, a tribe that is isolated by land that is eroding into the bay. It is also MY story—a public health nurse, born in Ohio, who traveled to Brazil as a Peace Corps volunteer in health and community development, to Virginia, to Texas, and finally to the Pacific Northwest. I reflect upon my own experiences, my culture, and my heritage as I am listening to and learning from members of the tribe. The chapters in this book are in three sections—my daily and monthly journal, cultural reflections, Native American and Celtic, and the lessons I learned simply by being present.

The stories are told using months of the Roman calendar as well as the times of the year as described by the tribe—when salmon run and berries bloom. Chapter headings are in English and Salish. The Salish is taken from the Quinault Council Annual Calendar. I begin my journey in September, or *Ts okwanpitskitl?lak* (leaves are getting red on the vine maples). I quote Native American leaders across North America. Their teaching is not only an exercise to improve tribal health, but to share with all peoples, that we all might heal from the illnesses that plague families and society. By taking these healing stories beyond the borders of the tiny land track of Cedar Bay I am reflecting something the tribal chairman said, "Even a small tribe has much to teach the world."

In the end, there is not one answer to the question of infant mortality—or even multiple answers. I hope that the reader reads between the lines the lessons that are found here. The answers to the questions concerning infant mortality may be in these stories, on this path and in these waters. This is a true story. It is told in a chronological calendar of fourteen months, starting with my first month and orientation to the closing ceremony. Please take the journey with me.

◆ ◆ ◆ ◆ ◆

Note: The five diamonds are an indication that I have transitioned time, location, or culture. I contrast or compare Native American culture with my own Celtic heritage. I draw upon memories of my own childhood, bringing in stories as they contribute to the awareness of cultural teachings.

There are no secrets.
There is no mystery.
There is only common sense.
—*Onondaga*

Words are the voice of the heart.
—*Tuscarora*

September

Ts okwanpitskitl?lak

Leaves are getting red on the vine maples

"We Will Teach the Nation"

The state supervisor referred me to the employee counseling service because she said I had a problem. I called for an appointment and took the first opening. It took the therapist exactly five minutes to determine my problem. He reached for his phone, spoke to the career transition center, and made a referral for me to see a career consultant that same day.

Sitting on the stone wall outside of the career transition center after office hours, the consultant presented a realm of possibilities. She was enthusiastic, hopeful, encouraging. This conversation led me to disengage from my Dilbert-like cubicle in the government bureaucracy, cutting the cord of security to my lucrative state job. At eight o'clock the next morning, I had an appointment with my doctor. I was on the edge. The work environment caused mental stress, and physically, my neck and shoulder muscles were frozen, and I could not reach the top shelf to put dishes away. When I stood up, my knees locked and cracked loudly. I needed to grab tabletops or chairs for support. At night, I slept with a rolled up pillow under my neck. Arthritis threatened to incapacitate me.

The doctor diagnosed my condition as "situational anxiety" and wrote a prescription: "Stay away from work for three weeks. Pursue a new job. Keep exercising." Prescription in hand, I left the doctor's office already feeling better. I reported to the career transition office where I had access to computers, counselors, newspapers, a library of books, and classes on "How to Interview," "Resume Writing," "Finding Your Chosen Career." I immersed myself. I wanted to be well.

One day, my career counselor handed me a four-line employment ad. A small Indian tribe in western Pacific County needed a project director. I sent my resume and a letter asking for an interview.

The Cedar Bay Indian Nation occupies a small tract of land in southern Washington where Willapa Bay meets the Pacific Ocean. There are approximately one hundred fifty people on the tribal membership rolls. On a dark, rainy evening in September, I drove to my interview at the reservation. Three weeks later the chairman of the tribe called me. He invited me to take the job, but asked that I carefully consider the offer because it was a three-year commitment, the life of the grant. Leaving before the grant was completed was unacceptable. Two days later, I accepted the position.

After committing to the tribe, I resigned from state service, cleaned out my desk, got my papers in order, and left at the end of the week. My friend Joyce, a state employee, nutritionist, and hiking buddy, remarked, "In your new job, you will heal."

The following Monday morning, I drove toward the Pacific Ocean. I stopped by the insurance office to let my agent know that I would be adding a longer commute to my car. The agent loaned me four books for the new job: *A Gathering of Wisdoms* by Swinomish Tribal Mental Health Project, *The Ancient Wisdom of the Medicine Wheel* by Roy Wilson, *Sacred Plant Medicine* by Stephen Harrod Buhner, and *Native American Rights* by D. Bender., B. Stalcup, and T. Roleff.

The Cedar Bay Tribal reservation is a two hour drive from my home in Olympia, Washington. Logging trucks outnumber passenger cars along the route.

My father taught me how to note my route. In the cavalry, he was trained to notice directions and take frequent looks back to see how the area would look if he returned by the same route. Here there are forests and clear cuts, a llama farm and the signs for an RV Park. I soon enter Harbor County, drive past small towns and exit for a break. I see a large mural on the side of a building depicting men with choker chains around a good-sized log. I fill my large mug with fresh coffee at a convenience store. When the attendant charges me a quarter, I decide that this will be my gas, coffee and rest stop from now on. I head south, past the local sawmill and lumber company where mountains of logs are stacked behind barbed wire. I drive past a mountain of sawdust and over a bridge. Full logging trucks pass me regularly. It's a tight fit. I drive past a tavern into the hills and hug the right lane, allowing the faster moving logging trucks to pass me.

I top a rise and begin the descent into town. Rotary signs, church signs, and "Welcome to Bryan" dot the side of the road. Rusted iron deer graze the top of the hill; a metal mother bear and her cubs meander across the grass—all part of Bryan's public art project. At the bottom of the hill, before the bridge into town, an intersecting route veers right at a yield sign. A large lumber mill hums away on the opposite side of the river. I take the turn and head west along the northern rim of Willapa Bay. Soon, a sign reads, "Reservation, 18 miles." The road proceeds across pasture land. I scan the fields for elk; a herd is occasionally seen in this area. The hills are clear-cut. I see no herd as the road winds and snakes toward the reservation. I learn later that Weyerhaeuser owns 90% of the forest in this area. I cross the bridge over North River, which empties into the Bay. I look for the eagle's nest that my co-worker Pat told me about. One day she saw both the eagle and the elk herd—good omens. I drive past men and trailers on the edge of the water. A green and white sign announces reservation land. A quarter of a mile later, I turn left onto Old Reservation Road. The speed limit is 25 miles per hour, "children nearby."

The tribal cemetery is on my left and the community center on my right, as I turn into the parking area. The Law Center, Tribal Court, and Chief of Police occupy the first building. Next to the Law Center is the Education Department. Behind the community center, a reddish canoe has seen better days. Beyond the canoe are the shoal waters, a mud flat area that fills and empties with the tides. The Pacific Ocean roars just around the bend.

I pause to take it all in. There is a presence here, a sense of connection. Remembering my summer church camp where the campers meditated silently in the woods before breakfast, I recall the Bible verse, "Be still, and know that I am God."

The tribal community center is a gathering place and a healing place. It houses the new clinic facility. There is a large dining room and kitchen to feed the seniors three times a week. It is a place of feasting and holidays. On the walls in the hallway to the dining area, murals depict two Northwest Indian legends, *Beaver Causes a Deluge* and *Mother Bore Puppies*. There are pictures of a field trip to the state capitol—children in big leather chairs in the Governor's Conference Room. Cupboards in the front lobby display masks. One of the masks is accompanied by a short story explaining what the painting of the mask means. From the lobby I walk into the large Tribal Community Meeting Room, named after the revered ancestral tribal community leader, Chief John Joseph Ta wal'a mish. On the north wall hang portraits of prominent tribe members from the past. Featured among these is Chief John Joseph, last of the Flatheads, a chief of royal heritage.

I go to the present day tribal chairman's office for orientation and then to receive my assignment from Chairman Thomas Greyhawk. He speaks of his deep love for the people and his commitment to making a difference in their lives. He explains my first assignment. I am to work with the women of the tribe, to empower them to gain knowledge to promote their own health care. They will in turn empower their families. The families in turn and in time will empower the community, which will become stronger and healthier. This cycle of wellness will spiral outward and expand to the native peoples in the county. From the county, wellness will spiral to the region.

The chairman explains the second assignment. The new health clinic, a beautiful state-of-the-art facility, must be owned by the tribal community. It is not to be a white-dominated clinic where the providers are one color serving people of another color. It was not to be a clinic of only one practice of medicine. It is to be a clinic that offers traditional and western practices of healing, a clinic to serve all people. The chairman is the director of the clinic. In the midst of changes and surrounded by dominant white culture, he wants the tribe to survive.

It is from this small tribe on this tiny reservation that I come to understand the ancient wisdom of the medicine wheel, the beautiful simplicity of the four directions of health—physical, mental, emotional and spiritual. East is the direction of new beginnings with the rising sun. Seeds are planted in the east and in the human life cycle; east represents the infant and child. South is warmth, growth, development and the fire of adolescence. West is reflection, the maturity of the adult and time to pause. North is white, the Elder who has wisdom.

Please, Grandfather, allow me to make a new beginning, to listen and learn with reverence and respect. Help me to contribute by sharing what I bring to this learning. Allow me to share. Let me be like the pebble that is tossed into the center of the pond. Let the understanding ripple outward.

◆ ◆ ◆ ◆ ◆

The scraggy looking area in this first photo was once forest. It has been clear-cut in my absence over a long holiday week-end. In time, plants will return and the land begin to green again. Life can return to the land.

Logs from the forest are taken to this mill where they are inventoried, tagged and guarded behind barbed wire fences—prisoners on their journey to foreign ports. One day on my commute, I count thirty-two logging trucks in two hours.

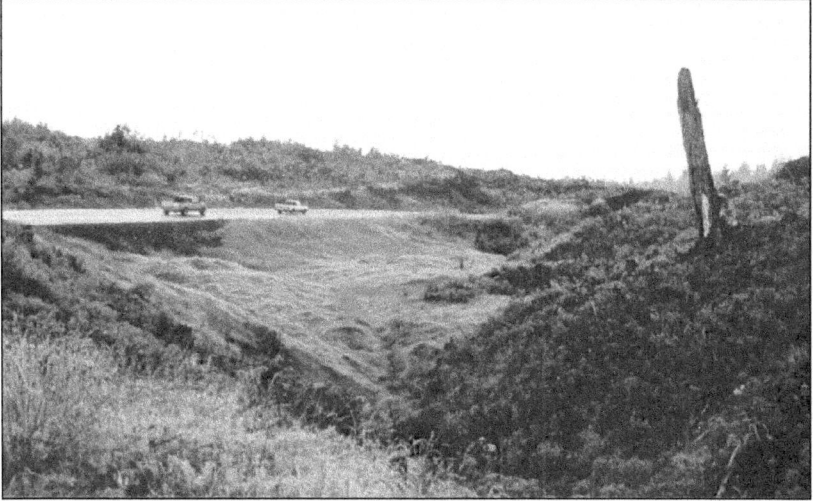

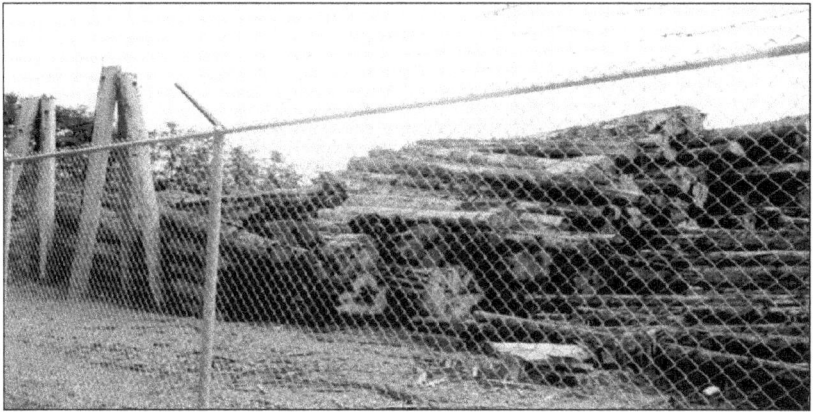

Leaves of Indian Tea

In the fall, not long after I began working with the tribe, my eldest daughter, a student at the University of Texas at Austin, called and told me she would be an usher at the memorial service for Congresswoman Barbara Jordan, who was a faculty member at UT. Barbara was one of my ideological, political and life mentors. She said, during a commencement address at Harvard in 1977:

> I don't know here, this afternoon, what will be next for me. I will not know what the next step is until I get there. I know that when I went to Boston, and Austin, and Washington, I took with me everything I had learned before. That is what I will do this time. That is the point of it, isn't it? To bring all you have with you wherever you go.

Barbara Jordon—the first black woman to serve Texas as a Congresswoman—spoke eloquently and forcefully from her wheelchair at the 1992 Democratic Convention. She called on the country to unite. Her work, done with honor, respect and hope, had earned her the Presidential Medal of Freedom.

Inspired by Jordon's quote, her struggles and her strong belief in the American Constitution, I take all that I am, all my experiences and even my stress and discomfort to the healing and wellness work on the reservation.

Although I went to the reservation with the expectation of directing a project to promote tribal health, my months in residence helped *me* to achieve *true* health. I learned the ancient wisdom of the medicine wheel— that all parts of the wheel are in balance, working in harmony, and this was to be *my* healing journey.

Many played a role in this healing journey: tribal elder Edith shared leaves of Indian Tea and sat patiently while I attempt to weave and stitch sweet grass and raffia baskets in the style that is traditional of the Chinook. A Tribal Board of Health member told me the story of listening. The mental health worker took time to listen to my story. Marge Potter, the community health representative who never spares words, handed me a copy of the book, *Native Wisdom for White Minds* by Ann Wilson Schaff. Edith George challenged me and taught me to be sensitive. Edith has other names in these chapters: The Elder, The Tribal Council Member, She-Who-Has-The-Same-Name, and finally, Buddy. In the end, Edith showed me how to transition the human and spiritual worlds. Chairman Greyhawk taught me lessons of leadership and what it is to be Indian in a white dominant culture. Descended from Chief John Joseph, he follows the wise and caring lead of his great-grandfather.

The state health department and the regional medical college were concerned with the high infant death rate within this tribal community. I was asked the same questions by many in the medical community: "What is the reason for the high infant mortality rate in the Cedar Bay Indian Tribe? Why are eleven out of nineteen pregnancies lost before term and why do two of the remaining live births end in death? Why are pregnancies ending prematurely?" Despite the frequency of the questions, I was dumbfounded by the implication that I was expected to have answers.

"We are a small tribe, but we have much to teach the world," the tribal chairman said on my first day at the reservation. Nine months later, the women of the circle, a focus planning group, agreed to make their stories public so that native women and non-native women could hear and heal from their individual pain. Four months after that, three women of this tribal community carried eleven original art story masks from the Pacific Coast to the Chesapeake Bay, to share their stories of loss, healing and hope. Upon return from Washington, D.C., the tribe's spiritual leader presented me with her mask; she instructed me to take "Spirit Mask" out into the world to be used for teaching.

Just fourteen months after the chairman's statement, the health access grant under which I was funded was terminated by the grant's advisors in Washington, D.C. The grant—which had been guaranteed for three-years—was ended prematurely, like the pregnancies on the reservation.

About the time that I was trying to decide if I should make public the stories of my journey with the tribe, I was nudged by a closing statement in a paper by one of the nursing students at the University of Washington. A registered nurse returning to the university to earn her bachelor's degree, this student worked on the surgical floor of the local hospital. An African/American, she was struggling, alone in a sea of white faces and uniforms. For her independent study, which I was supervising, she was reading literature by black nurses. Her project paper closed with these two questions:

"Will I be able to speak up for social justice? Will you?" As if the questions were directed to me personally, I wondered if I had the courage to speak to the social injustices that I encountered on the tribal reservation? Could I provide an image of social injustice that contributes to dominant culture understanding?

I considered what I had endured alongside the tribe—the politics of the grant, the barriers to communication with a funding source across the country and the meager budget for the project. The national advisors group was impressive: top doctors of the Centers for Disease Control, the American Medical Association, the Federal Department of Disease and Infection Control and the Environmental Protection Agency, flew to Washington State and met at the airport to discuss the needs of the tribe— but did not actually visit the reservation. An evaluation team of four representing the Robert Wood Johnson Foundation and the Kaiser Foundation did come to the tribe in February of 1996—a diverse cultural representation of Chinese, West Indian, Native American and African/American. The tribal women looked forward to this visit and prepared by beading necklaces for gifts and roasting salmon. When the four arrived, they had little time to hear the stories of the women; they instead asked questions because they needed responses for their reports. Where was the commitment to bridge barriers of communication, to listen? The evaluation team paused briefly in their process when the women of the tribe stepped forward to offer their gifts of appreciation for coming to the reservation.

This tribe has often been exploited by white journalists and university researchers, but after writing their bylines and completing their surveys, few returned to listen and hear the stories of the tribal members. Only one group is remembered by the tribe as listening. They were a group of student nurses. These nursing students who had originally failed in their tribal diabetes education project returned a second time to listen, revise their work, and put it into the language of the tribe. They left a program that continues to be used for tribal education today.

During the course of my project, I experienced resistance from many quarters, including politicians, foundation administrators and even tribal members. Will I have the courage to return to the issues that are barriers to communication?

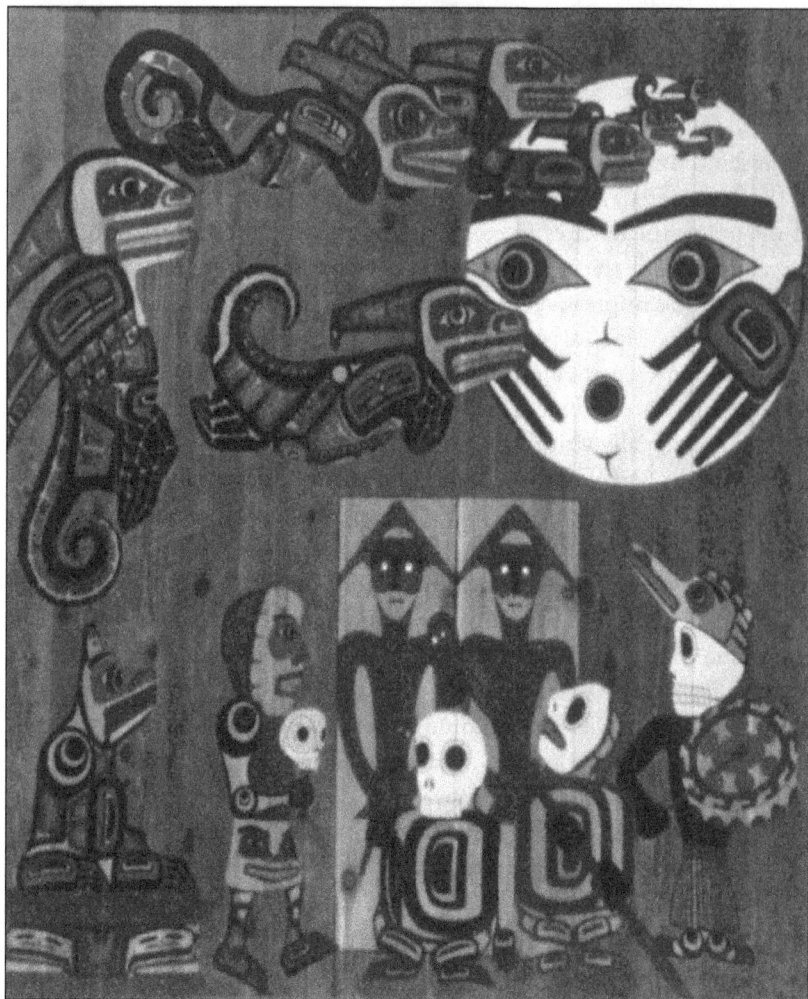

This large cedar board painting by artist Tom Anderson hangs on the south wall of the Tribal Community Meeting Room at the Long House and Tribal Community Center and Clinic of the Cedar Bay Indian Nation. It is named "Trail of the Spirits" or "Untitled." The ancient watchers with their shaman sticks look down upon the gathered.

Headlines

Federal probe of Cedar Bay infant mortality under way....

A tribe's babies are dying—and no one knows why.

Losing a whole generation. Study probes puzzle of tribe's infant deaths....

Cedar Bay Tribe wracked by deaths....

Cedar Bay gets federal help only after 15 of 23 are lost....

A People in Crisis. Tribe: wants to open own health clinic....

Cedar Bay Tribe will bury another baby. Indian tribe is losing infants to medical mystery....

Concerned leaders declared a medical emergency and asked state health officials to intervene....

Babies: Tribe's poverty and isolation are cited....

Diabetes rate high among members of Cedar Bay Tribe....

Indians: Doctor found undiagnosed incidence of hepatitis at reservation....

The above headlines were written during the health emergency declared in 1992.

In June 1996, a journalist from *The Seattle Times* returned to Cedar Bay for an update. The resulting article began:

The Cedar Bay Tribe Rides into the Next Century. Sequestered by whites, ravaged by smallpox, plagued by infant deaths and harassed by an aggressive Pacific Ocean, the state's smallest native tribe has endured the unthinkable and seeks the improbable: to survive and thrive into the next millennium.

The Joint Report by Cedar Bay Indian Tribe, Indian Health Service and the University of Washington states:

> The Tribe's concern about high rates of adverse outcomes of on-reservation pregnancies between 1988-1992 was corroborated by the data. Nineteen pregnancies were identified; none ended in a voluntary termination of pregnancy. Although the rates were based on small numbers and therefore unstable, the rates and ratios help document the severity of the problem of adverse outcomes of the on-reservation pregnancies, compared with the "expected" rate.

Why? What was the reason for the high rate of infant mortality? Washington State Congresswoman Jolene Unsoeld sought funding for the problem. This tiny Indian tribe on the West Coast, much smaller in number than many family reunions, received the nation's top advisors.

October

Pan?silpaulos

Time of Autumn

The Daily Log

In this new job, I wanted to feel part of the team in the workplace and to understand the tribal community and that it was okay to be here. To boost my confidence, I kept a log of my activities and what I learned, a record that helped me track.

October 16—Time of preparation for winter

Orientation. Meet with the tribal chairman. Sign papers. Learn computer entry. Lunch in the dining room after the elders are served.

October 17

Meet personnel in the main building and the educational building. Begin discussions with personnel concerning their work as it relates to the grant I am directing. Try to relax and allow the information to seep in.

October 18

I am tired. I have been looking for local housing but not finding anything. I walk out of the store, get into my car and head up the coast.

October 19

I meet with the tribal police officer. He looks like he can handle trouble, but I get the feeling he is a gentle person. He tells me his family resides on the Nez Perce Reservation in Eastern Washington and Idaho. He is Chippewa by birth and comes from a closed reservation in Minnesota.

"What is closed?" I ask him.

"Only three reservations in the United States are closed. At the time of President Lincoln, a closed reservation meant that the whites were not allowed on the property. Today, whites are still not allowed on the property. Only whites who are employees on the reservation may come and go

33

to their work, but they may not loiter or otherwise be on the reservation."

The tribal mental health counselor, the community health representative and I go out to lunch. We drive ten miles up the coast to the nearest town. Over lunch, we decide to invite a Native American public health nurse to hold a health promotion talking circle and to invite her to lead a sweat, which is a healing circle in a sweat lodge. Later that same day, the community health representative introduces me around the reservation. This is a good day.

October 20

I talk with the tribal administrator about the population served by the clinic. There are about 150 tribal members on the membership rolls. Fifty members live in close proximity to the health clinic. Tribal children attend schools in the neighboring county because those schools are closer to the reservation. A school bus picks up and returns children to the reservation.

October 23

The ancient language of the Cedar Bay is called *Ta wal' a mish.* The historical trade language of the area, however, is of the Chinook nation. Cultures prominent to the heritage of Cedar Bay are Lower Chehalis, Lower Chinook and Quinault, and to a lesser degree, the Nisqually, Puyallup, and other ancestors who traded in these regions. The tribes of the Northwest were smaller family groups who inhabited the rivers and coast. Since marriage in the same family group was taboo, tribes often traded (or stole) wives. A native friend in the Department of Social and Health Services once told me that all Washington State Native Americans are related. The Cedar Bay tribe are descended from the Canoe People. Because of their location on the river, bay and coast, they did their visiting, ceremonies, food gathering and fishing by canoe.

Related stories: my friend, who is of Cowlitz heritage, went to an American school. At the end of the day, he reviewed the school lessons with his medicine woman grandmother. She re-taught him the lessons in the Indian way. Being Indian is attitude as well as bloodline. Another friend of Quinault heritage told me how the federal government divided Indian lands and gave ownership to each member. Many Indians, accustomed to common ownership, sold off their parcels. Reservations became checkerboards of Indian and non-Indian ownership. Once off the land, the Indians had no place to go.

October 24

Today, I visit the Washington Room of the State Library in Olympia, far from the reservation. Several cabinets are stocked with copies of historic legal cases involving fishing rights and use of forested lands. Historical and ancestral use of common land and the use of the sea gave way to constant struggles over lumber companies' use of the forests and the multi-national use of fishing rights on the seas and rivers. There are many more mouths to feed and much profit involved. Land and water use is very complicated and transcends many national, cultural and economic issues. During a break in my review, I pick a book from a shelf and the first page leaps out at me. Written by a white author concerning the education of Native Peoples, it speaks of the need to re-locate native children to boarding schools for proper education. "We must educate these heathens."

What must it be like to be told that everything your grandparents taught was wrong, that you could not speak your own language and that you must learn proper domestic skills? I can not imagine denying everything my beloved grandfather taught me.

October 25

The health contract supervisor was discussing health care payment plans with me when a young pregnant tribal woman comes into the tribal clinic to apply for prenatal care. She needs to be referred to the state's First Steps program, which serves low income and high risk pregnancies. She has few choices about her medical care, and can either travel eighteen miles to the south to a community clinic or forty-five miles north to a community hospital. Access to obstetrical care involves not only the choice of provider, but finding transportation to get to the provider. It involves education about nutrition, prenatal care management and, because of the history of fetal loss, close monitoring of environmental factors as well.

October 26

It is still misty as I drive along the outer bank of the harbor. Several of the fishing boats have already left port. I am on schedule but still thinking I need to leave ten minutes earlier in order to sign in at the reservation desk by 8:30 a.m. Today, I pull out of the garage at 7:04 because I have an early morning swim workout at the "Y." Swimming puts things into perspective for me and relieves my aching joints. I have been feeling stiff lately. Could be age related, which I do not want to admit. Denial. That's what it is. Just keep swimming, arm over arm and get into the swim of things at the "rez" as well.

On the road ahead, I see a herd of cattle crossing. The farmer hustles the last few as I down-shift. As I pass, the herder waved.

I sign in at the front desk seven minutes late. There is to be a tribal meeting and I wonder if I will be introduced. I head to the center annex, a half-mile down the road, for an appointment with Roberto, the shellfish biologist and economic developer for the tribe's oyster company. He tells me about chemicals used to kill spartina, a cord grass that chokes seeding oysters. Spartina comes from the east coast with eastern oyster seeds and now is growing out of control in the bay, clogging the tidewaters. Willapa is the largest producing bay for oysters in the country. The tribal company is one of eleven oyster producers which lay their seedbeds in and harvest oysters from what is known as "the most pristine bay in the country."

Roberto continued, "The tribe is encouraging other commercial oyster harvesters to control spartina by natural methods." He opposes using the commercial chemical *Seven* because he thinks it is carcinogenic. Roberto explains, "Ghost or burrowing shrimp are also consuming our oyster seeds. The once prevalent sturgeon and coho salmon historically consumed ghost shrimp. Ghost shrimp form a u-shaped tube and create large holes in the oyster beds. *Seven* is used to kill the ghost shrimp, but at the same time it is polluting the bay."

October 27

Today, I meet with the environmental program manager. "Surfactants are used by Weyerhaeuser to kill insects in the forests," she explains. "Undergrowth must be kept down to allow more sun, helping the commercial trees grow faster." Forests surround the reservation. "Any chemical spray used in the forest could conceivably waft across the residential neighborhoods of the reservation."

She begins to list the problems: "Fecal matter left by cows wading through the near-by streams and rivers is a concern because this is a source of E. coli."

"This area is like a tree farm. There are no old growth or big trees left; it is all private forest with none owned by the tribe," she continues.

I have passed eight loaded logging trucks barreling down the road to the Port. Only one was carrying finished lumber; the only truck that had been to a local sawmill.

Two weeks before, a full logging truck struck a car carrying two high school students. The girls were on their lunch break and driving on the wrong side of the road. The truck swerved to avoid the car. The car swerved to avoid the truck. I now see white crosses on the side of the road during my commute. The community is in shock and deep grief.

October 30

The environmental program manager is conducting water quality tests for the next two days. Five officials from the Environmental Protection Agency in Seattle are at the tribal center to test the water samples they collected on the reservation and in close proximity to the reservation. A table is placed at the door of the center, and elaborate equipment is set up. One of the tests is for mercury. The testers draw a sample from water that had been sitting in the pipes overnight. If mercury is present, it will most likely appear in the first water sample of the morning.

The experts, with the help of Roberto, discuss chemicals, using a map that shows the proximity of residences to the water sources and streams and run-off on the beaches. The community health worker shows me the commercial bottled water on her desk. The physician's assistant and his wife spend about forty dollars per month on bottled water. I consider the number of cups of coffee I drink from the community coffee pot, which is brewed with tap water. I decide to limit my daily intake to one cup. There remain a lot of unanswered questions concerning water quality.

November 1—A time of harvest and thanksgiving

Roberto says he is one-half Mexican. "I am Aztec, but that doesn't count for anything here." I tell him I am of the McGregor Clan of the northern highlands of Scotland, but I do not think that counts for anything either.

At lunch, the elders are fed first, out of respect. If there is anything left, the staff can eat for $1.50. The meal includes green salad, purple cole slaw, red chili beans with grated cheddar cheese and freshly diced onions, baked potato halves and ground beef. I add butter and chives to the potatoes. The smell of the brownies leads me to the dessert table. I sit and look out windows facing the tidewaters of the Pacific.

In the afternoon, the community health worker guides me in a neighborhood door-to-door introduction to the tribal families. She has a list of residents and tribal members, which I study to understand family relationships.

On my way home, I pick up my new business cards.

November 2

The EPA finished testing. I wonder if it is okay to continue drinking coffee. The chairman comes into my office and pulls up a chair. We discuss the importance of a women's health focus group. He gently but firmly directs me to concentrate my work on supporting the women who have lost infants and on analyzing the tribe's access to reproductive care in general.

November 3

Today the tribal leadership, clinic staff and I meet with the administrative and clinic leadership of the county health department. We make plans to share our health programs and resources. An important collaboration begins.

November 4

I review an assessment survey with the education director and the director of the mental health program. Then, I meet with the environmental program manager to get the results from the water quality test. "It will take two months to get the results," she says.

I decide to continue drinking coffee, brewed with tribal waters, for another two months. As I turn to leave her office, I see paper art by the file cabinets—a structure of bamboo poles to which a large sheet of paper has been attached by wrapping the paper around the pole frame. Leather straps have been used to lace the paper to the poles. The paper is made from spartina grass and is earthy, rough, and various shades of brown. One area of the paper has a dark flat reed woven into it. At the top of the paper are inked these words of Chief Sealth, also known as Chief Seattle:

> All things are
> bound together.
> What happens
> to the earth happens
> to the children of
> earth.
> Man has not woven
> the well of life.

He is but one thread.
Whatever he does,
he does to himself.

I consider the use of spartina grass as paper, and wonder how it weaves. Hazel Pete of the Chehalis tribe uses natural earthen materials for her baskets. Perhaps this invasive weed can be woven into something functional and beautiful.

The wind is blowing hard outside, picking up rain over the tidewaters and tossing it horizontally over the land.

The environmental program manager has a six-month old son who is healthy and developing well. I ask her about the obstetrical care she received. She was employed, had adequate health care coverage, and her car was in good repair. She chose to travel eighty miles to see a female obstetrician. Other women on the reservation do not have the same choices. Tribal women have to take whatever health care is available under Indian Health Service guidelines, and this care is available only as long as allocated money was not used up by someone's sudden illness. There are many women on the reservation with inadequate health care, cars in disrepair, and homes isolated by icy roads in winter.

It is 4:30 p.m. and the coastal storm is intensifying. I anticipate a power outage, a frequent occurrence.

November 7

I begin the day with my own health care by visiting the dentist. It has been three years since I have been in the dental chair. As a result, the hygienist needs to take a chisel to the tartar. I recall a scene from years earlier:

◆ ◆ ◆ ◆ ◆

I remember the Brazilian Pantenal, a wildlife refuge located in the western part of Brazil, near the geographic center of South America. My youngest daughter Susan, then eight years old, accompanied me for a visit to the town where I had been a volunteer public health nurse with the Peace Corps. With a guide and his truck, we headed into alligator—*carangeju*—country. From a good vantage point some distance away, we saw the alligators open their big mouths while a small black bird picked and cleaned their teeth. These birds were alligator hygienists and the symbiotic relationship between them was one of respect and tolerance.

◆ ◆ ◆ ◆ ◆

The morning fog has burned off. The drive to the reservation is crisp and colorful. There are as many logging trucks on the roads as I usually see earlier in the day. Where do they all come from?

November 8

I attend a Partnership meeting at the county seat. Funded by the Washington State Legislature under the Public Health Improvement Plan, this is a gathering of community leaders and agencies to address general health issues for the entire county. The first order of business is to mourn the two high school students who were killed by the logging truck.

November 10

I leave for my own professional gathering, the American Public Health Association annual meeting in San Diego. At previous annual meetings I attended maternal and child health and tuberculosis sessions. This year, I will attend sessions on Native American health.

November 16

This is the fourth week of my assignment; time has passed quickly. Everyone has left the building except me. All staff supported by federal dollars have gone because of a mandated federal shutdown. The federal budget has not been passed. The clinic is closed. The dental office is locked. Only project people are left. It is no fun to work in an empty building. Nancy, the clinic's medical assistant, went to the unemployment office and found the lines so long that she returned home. The community health worker is at home. She is my most important advisor, and I could make all kinds of tribal faux pas without her. The local newspaper states "The federal shutdown makes no difference. Workers will be paid, regardless. Services will go on as usual." That is not the case on the reservation.

November 18

Although she does not get a paycheck with the health clinic closed, the mental health counselor comes back to work anyway. She was hired because of her experience working with abused and grieving clients. I tell her of the break-up with my boyfriend of two years. "You must feel a loss," she responds. I sit with her and cry.

December 1

After trying several possibilities, I find a place within the community to stay—a room in a compact cedar log cabin, known as a pan-abode—two miles down the road from the tribal center. The owner keeps a wood fire burning all night, stoking and adding a wood at about 4:00 a.m. The woman's ninety-year-old piano-playing mother died last year, leaving this room available for guests. The full-sized bed is covered with a lovely family heirloom quilt. When I feel the warmth of the log stove, see the piano complete with song book, and notice that a black dachshund, Pepper, has already secured her spot in front of the stove, I settle in for Ms. Marian's Greek hospitality.

December 21

I am learning more of the logistics and the mechanics of this place. When will I begin to feel a part of the life of this community? I have one daughter in Texas, another in Oregon, and my youngest is finishing her senior year in Olympia, which is one reason I commute these roads—back and forth, back and forth—twice weekly. Monday to the reservation and Ms. Marian's for an overnight. Tuesday night, home to Olympia. Wednesday morning, back to the reservation. The weeks go like that.

December 28

The day begins with a staff meeting. The discussion includes the idea of developing a woman's health clinic to serve the Indian people of the entire county. I am particularly interested in this, and do my best to participate and sound informative. After the staff meeting, I am taken aside by one of the members of the Tribal Board of Health who courteously asks if he might speak with me. I sense that I have not been sensitive or might have violated protocol in some way. We choose a quiet room and the board of health member begins to tell me a story, the traditional way of teaching. My heart is beating, expecting a reprimand. I want to shout in my Yankee way, "Don't beat around the bush. Tell me directly what I did wrong so that I can get it right!" However, I keep quiet and listen. No reprimand comes, and the story continues. I relax and listen. He tells me of a meeting he once had with the tribal chairman. Their discussion focused on ideas for conducting a future program. He felt he had many good ideas and knew just how the program should be conducted, and yet he chose to remain quiet. Then, the chairman himself introduced the very ideas that he would have brought to the discussion. In this way, he knew that his ideas would have support. When the story is finished, I thank him for taking the time to teach me. That evening after work, I drive back to the cedar pan-abode.

After dinner, as Ms. Marian watched Vanna turn over the letters on Wheel of Fortune, I excuse myself and go to my room. Tucking the wool blanket and her mother's quilt snugly under my chin, I ponder the story. As I drift off to sleep, I begin to understand. Even though I have valuable information from the state health office and even though I have some good answers and perhaps great suggestions, I should listen and receive what I need from the tribe. I am to listen to the wisdom of the chairman, their leader. I am to listen to the women who have suffered loss. All that I bring to this work will be used in time. All that I need to heal will be provided. It is all here.

January 10

The wife of the tribal chairman stops by my office to chat. She is the tribal religious leader. Her own Lummi tribe is farther north, on Puget Sound. Members of her family tribe often come to the reservation to support religious, healing, and celebration ceremonies. After she leaves my office, I jot down a poem, inspired by her story of braiding the chairman's hair every morning.

With This Hair

Father, Son and Holy Spirit
Father, Son and Holy Spirit
Father, Son and Holy Spirit

As the smooth long hair of the chairman
is divided into thirds and neatly braided into one

the prayer is silent, unspoken
as his wife guides the strands into place

The chairman fidgets
anxious to begin a new day's work at the tribal center
"Be still," she admonishes. *"I am praying."*

The chairman obeys, and she continues to the end.

Father, Son and Holy Spirit
Father, Son and Holy Spirit
Father, Son and Holy Spirit

A new day begins on the reservation

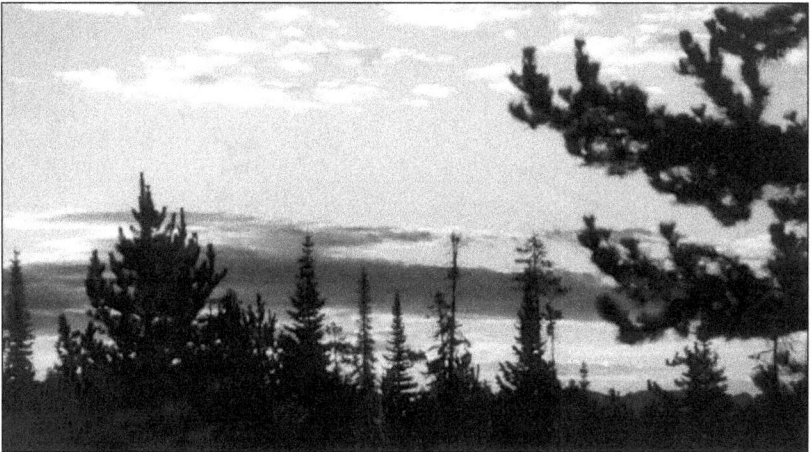

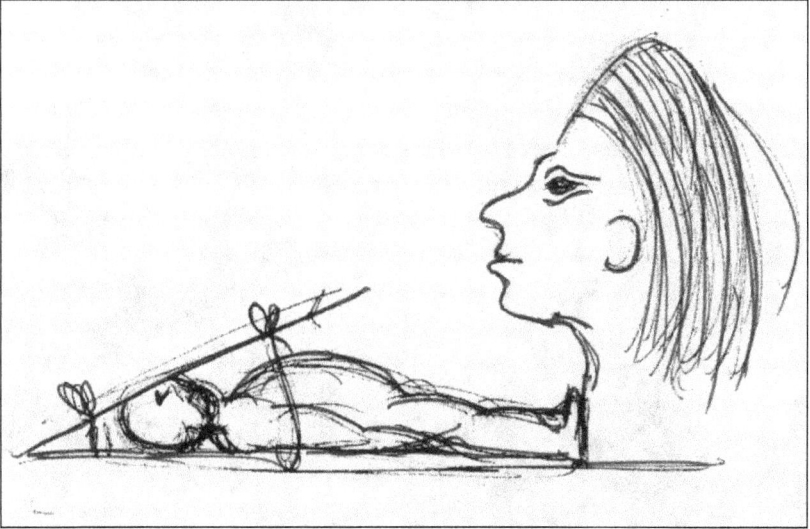

sketch by the author

The Ancestral Chief

A gallery of family portraits hangs on the wall of the tribal meeting room. Prominent among the portraits of the ancestors is an oil portrait of Chief John Joseph Tawalamish.

I sit under the portrait and look up into the face of a reddish-brown skinned man with a flat forehead under a headband of feathers. I am staring at a portrait of one recognized by both the native and non-native population surrounding the tribe as a great humanitarian. Chief John Joseph is the father, grandfather, great grandfather and great uncle of many of the current Cedar Bay tribal members. The father of John Joseph was a leader of the Cedar Bay band of Lower Chehalis Indians who were granted this reservation in 1855. His father saw to it that his son as an infant had his head bound to the cradleboard in the traditional fashion which was a sign of royal heritage. This special infant child was the last in his tribe to receive this practice.

Chief John Joseph is honored and loved by the people of Willapa Bay. His spirit pervades the small reservation. It is reported that even though Chief John Joseph was not physically a large man, he walked taller and straighter than anyone else. He had a quiet dignity and authority that everyone felt. He was invaluable to the white fishing company as he told them where and when to seine salmon. The process of seining is dropping a net in a half-moon circle and then pulling it to shore with horses. As the net tightens, the salmon struggle with great strengh to return to the water. Horses and men tug at the net to pull the bulk to shore until the entire net rests above the water. The plentiful catch was credited to the knowledge of the chief, passed down to him through many generations. A story is told by a non-native community member who was eight years old at the time.

> In the summer time when I was not in school, I tagged along after my father to watch the seining of the salmon down at the dock not far from the tribal reservation. I got to be with the Chief as he worked so softly and with authority and knowledge among all the seiners. The

45

Chief was a man who was respected by all who knew him, no matter what race or color. He had assumed leadership of his small band of Indians and he worked valiantly on their behalf even though it seemed so sad that they did not advance. But, I want to tell you how he affected me and what I learned from him.

Occasionally we had visitors to the seining. One day, a man brought a 30-30 rifle, and I watched as the men took turns shooting at seals, which were just outside the surf line, treading water with only their heads and shoulders above the water surface. The seals were there every day, lining up for hours to watch, it seemed to me, the strange fishing practices of the humans. I was offered the chance to hold the rifle and shoot. I took that chance hoping for a pat on the back. My shot landed not on target but within a few feet of the baby seals that were following the adults. Wanting a response from my elders, I looked over my shoulder to see Chief John Joseph walking toward us all on the beach. He stopped a few feet away, and slowly turned his eyes from me to each man in turn. He said nothing. I was silent. The men became silent. I could feel tension mount, and then dissipate. The Chief turned and walked away. The rifle's owner unloaded his rifle. The seals were never bothered the rest of that summer, but an even more powerful lesson was learned in the silence of no words. Men were not to kill the animals for sport alone.

It is an unspoken and unwritten law. It is the understood principle of our relationship with the animals.

Since I have come to work at the reservation, there have been occasions when I have been told stories. I think about the story and dig for the lesson. I consider this method of teaching as I stand, lecture style, in front of my students and realize they might learn better through stories as well. I ask the student nurses to gather in a circle to tell stories of home visits with families in the community. Their peers listen intently. "We learn from the stories," they say.

In 1935, a local newspaper reported Chief John Joseph's passing.

While fishing alone with a dip net at the mouth of the Quinault River....

In all history, the commitment to sacrifice oneself for the people has been the definitive element of true human greatness; by that measure, John Joseph Tawalamish surely ranks as one of the great Indian chiefs.

The Chinooks, ancient masters of both land and sea when Lewis and

Clark came more than 200 years ago, believed that salmon were one form of ancestral reincarnation, sent to them each year from a mysterious home far from shore. Another belief was that the salmon's skeleton, particularly the backbone, must be thrown in the river to provide a form for their spirits on the return to the ocean. I have a dim memory of Chief John Joseph, at our Tree Island barbecues, tossing the salmon spines into the falling tide....

I must believe that, as the great wave engulfed his body off the shore, the spirit of John Joseph was borne away by the salmon people, and he became one with them on the way to their far and secret place in the dark, deep rolling sea.

Farewell, my Chief....

November

Panitpuhtuhkstista

Time when the clouds are covering

Assessment

I ponder about the reason for the high rate of infant mortality. Could it be history, heritage, local business practices or lack of adequate and timely access to health care? Can modern medical practice fix it? Can I as a nurse do something to help?

My brother calls me from New Jersey to ask a similar question concerning the tribe. He read about the Cedar Bay health emergency in the *Wall Street Journal.* "What is Washington state doing to its Indian populations?" Since I am working with the tribe, my brother as well as others in the dominant culture think that because I am here, I should have answers to these questions.

A few residents from the southern part of the county recognize that they are connected to the tribe by water and land. They also know that the concerns of the tribe reach beyond the boundaries of the reservation. County public health nurses working the areas bordering the reservation report that the number of miscarriages and infant anomalies found among their caseloads has increased.

As I delve into their reports, what should I ask? Are the causes behind a high infant death rate in the environment, lack of access to quality health care providers, chronic disease, economics, nutrition, alcohol and substance abuse, spirit sickness, soul loss, eroding land, poverty, dominant society indifference, fear of annihilation, politics?

I re-read *Ancient Wisdom of the Medicine Wheel* by Roy Wilson, after which I meet with the chairman. He explains to me, "The medicine wheel teaches that there must be a balance of the physical, mental, emotional, and spiritual aspects of health. If any one of the four is out of balance, then the whole is not healthy. Within that wheel are other factors that affect health, such as economic, educational, and nutritional." I can see that on this reservation, there is an imbalance. The wheel is not a circle. It is a lopsided melon. The spokes are uneven or broken, distorting the shape and compromising the strength of the wheel.

In 1994, the Washington state legislature passed the Public Health Improvement Plan (PHIP), a blueprint for improving the health of Washington citizens through prevention and improved access to care. The plan was based on specific objectives and requirements of the Health Services Act of 1993: control health system costs, ensure universal access to needed health services for all state residents and improve the health of the state's population. From the PHIP: "The Public Health Improvement Plan has three components: Assessment, Policy Development and Quality Assurance or Evaluation. The first component, Assessment, is the regular collection, analysis, and sharing of information about health conditions, risks, and resources in a community. Assessment activities identify trends in illness, injury and health and the factors that may cause these events."

November is devoted to assessment. The program I am directing will use the Medicine Wheel to assess the status of the physical, mental, emotional and spiritual health of tribal members. We will then develop programs to meet identified needs, and then evaluate the effectiveness of those programs. As the program is evaluated, so will it begin assessment again. The circular process is ongoing. The implemented programs change and adapt as more information is gained from the evaluation. It begins to spiral outward to community.

All this sounds academic and political. In theory, all Washington residents have the right to access quality health care, and this quality and the nature of the access must be regularly evaluated. A special memo from the secretary of health stated that Indians would be "at the table;" that Native Americans would NOT be left out of health care. Something about this basic right has been denied.

The tribal environmental program manager maps out for me the areas in close proximity to the reservation. Her map shows the surrounding forests, locations of cranberry fields where pesticides are used, failed septic systems with toxic materials that leach into the soil, the location of the burrowing bay shrimp, spartina cord grass in the bay and also the shellfish collection area.

I begin to realize the interconnection of the environment with the tribe and the agencies commissioned to protect the environment and the people within. The map is filled with these connections. I place the map in my office for easy reference. At times, I take the sheet from the wall, roll it up and carry it to a nursing class to discuss environmental health and its relation to maternal and child health.

At a meeting of faculty and public health nurse practitioners, the speaker discusses the Hanford nuclear plant on a toxic waste cleanup list. I begin to formulate questions. Might there be a connection between Hanford's nuclear waste and the reservation? In what direction does the toxic waste flow? Do the toxins in the water cause genetic changes? Might fish from toxic waters harm a woman planning to conceive? Might consumption of contaminated fish damage a developing fetus?

I attend the fall potluck dinner of the International Club at South Puget Sound Community College. I am a host mother to a student from Japan. While eating stir-fry and noodles, one of the other housemothers relates a story she watched on public television. Genetic changes, she reports, were noted in fish from the Willamette River. The Willamette runs into the Columbia River near Portland. It is downstream from the Hanford plant on the Washington side and upstream from the Trojan nuclear plant on the Oregon side. She asks me what I know of nuclear waste and water contamination. Without answering out loud, my mind begins to take an inventory of what I know about possible toxic contamination.

I know of dead birds.

Stopping by the tribal grocery, I overhear the story of a local resident who gathered her family and moved from the area in order to complete her pregnancy closer to the city medical clinic and further from the tidewaters. She and her children had been walking on the beach not far from the reservation lands when they came upon a flock of dead birds.

I know of dead crabs.

The chemical dependency counselor relates another mysterious story. While walking his dog on the beach north of the reservation, he witnessed thousands of Dungeness crab, some clinging to the trees and bushes, others flung up on the beach. Whole, healthy-looking crabs. All dead. He abandoned his walk.

I know of side effects from chemicals used for noxious plants.

At a New Year's Eve party, I meet one of the cranberry farmers whose fields lie north of the reservation. He told me about the industry and how chemicals are used to keep down unwanted growth.

I know of chemicals used in the nearby forests.

Spraying of undergrowth in the forests is done to provide more sunlight to spur faster growth of trees that will be sent to market.

I know of frog mutations.

A friend sent me a newspaper clipping which shows a genetically deformed frog from a contaminated lake in Wisconsin. The right leg of the frog had two feet.

I know of research in the Florida Everglades.

The front page of the local paper featured the story of a visiting professor from Florida. Dr. Louis Gillette shared his research from eight years working with alligators in the Florida Everglades. The alligators' reproductive systems had been genetically altered, his research showed. His evidence pointed strongly to the fertilizer plant upstream.

Meanwhile, the EPA water quality report arrives. There are no appreciable amounts of contaminants in the residential water supplies and there is no lead in the pipes. The bacteria count is not above acceptable levels. Even with that information, water filters donated by a naturopathic physician are installed in each home on the reservation.

I continue to ask myself questions. What does appreciable amounts mean? What are the government standards? On what are those standards based? Are all populations treated the same?

On a fresh flip chart page in my office, I sketch the distances from the tribal center to health care providers in the area. There are good two-lane roads to all facilities and providers. The roads along the coast and through the mountains can be treacherous on stormy winter nights but provide a pleasant, beautiful drive in the summer. Ten miles north up the Pacific coast, a physician's assistant staffs the closest clinic. The next town, fifteen miles away, has a clinic staffed by a doctor of osteopathy and a nurse practitioner. The next town is forty-five miles from the reservation and has obstetricians and a community hospital.

To the east is the state capital where there are two large hospitals. The drive from the reservation is approximately two hours. An alternative route from the reservation takes you along the northern rim of the bay and through the forest. This is a beautiful drive in the summer months, but is treacherous with black ice in the winter.

A visit to a health care practitioner is a major output in energy, expense, and time for tribal members, and is dependent upon adequate transportation. At the time of the health emergency in 1992, the tribe felt isolated and distant from the care centers.

Access to medical care is one problem, but there are additional barriers. Some tribal women believe that an attitude of prejudice exists in both the non-native and the native cultures toward their families. When they perceive prejudice, fear, or ignorance on the part of a provider, they often did not speak out. They simply do not return to the provider and seek alternative care.

I begin to visit area health care providers. I want to understand their beliefs and attitudes in serving Native American clients as well as to understand what the health care provider's needs are in relating to and caring for native women.

The tribal chairman envisions a medical conference to be held at the tribal center that would bring area health care providers together to share in the life and ceremony of the community. Such an event might help break down barriers between the non-native provider community and the native community.

One of my visits is to a nurse practitioner and shaman, who is on staff at the clinic to the southeast of the reservation. He combines his western nursing education with Indian traditional healing. At the end of our discussion about tribal health and speculations on infant mortality, he pulls from his bag a bracelet of tightly woven one-eighth inch cedar strips. In making this bracelet, the cedar bark was gathered in the traditional way—requesting permission from the spirit of the tree that the bark might be used for healing. He gives me the bracelet as a gift. This woven cedar bracelet connects me with the sacred cedar tree, firmly rooted to the earth.

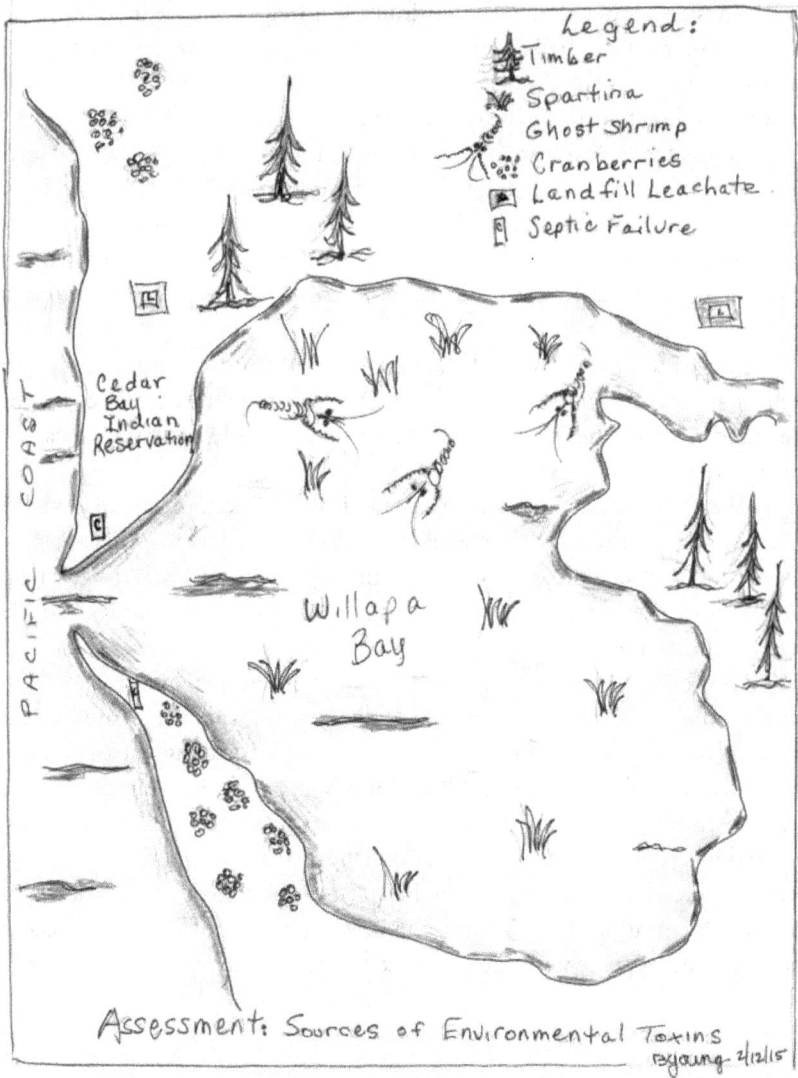

Legend:
- Timber
- Spartina
- Ghost Shrimp
- Cranberries
- Landfill Leachate
- Septic Failure

Cedar Bay Indian Reservation

PACIFIC COAST

Willapa Bay

Assessment: Sources of Environmental Toxins

Byoung- 2/12/15

Sketch of environmental toxins as taught to me by the director of the tribal environmental program.

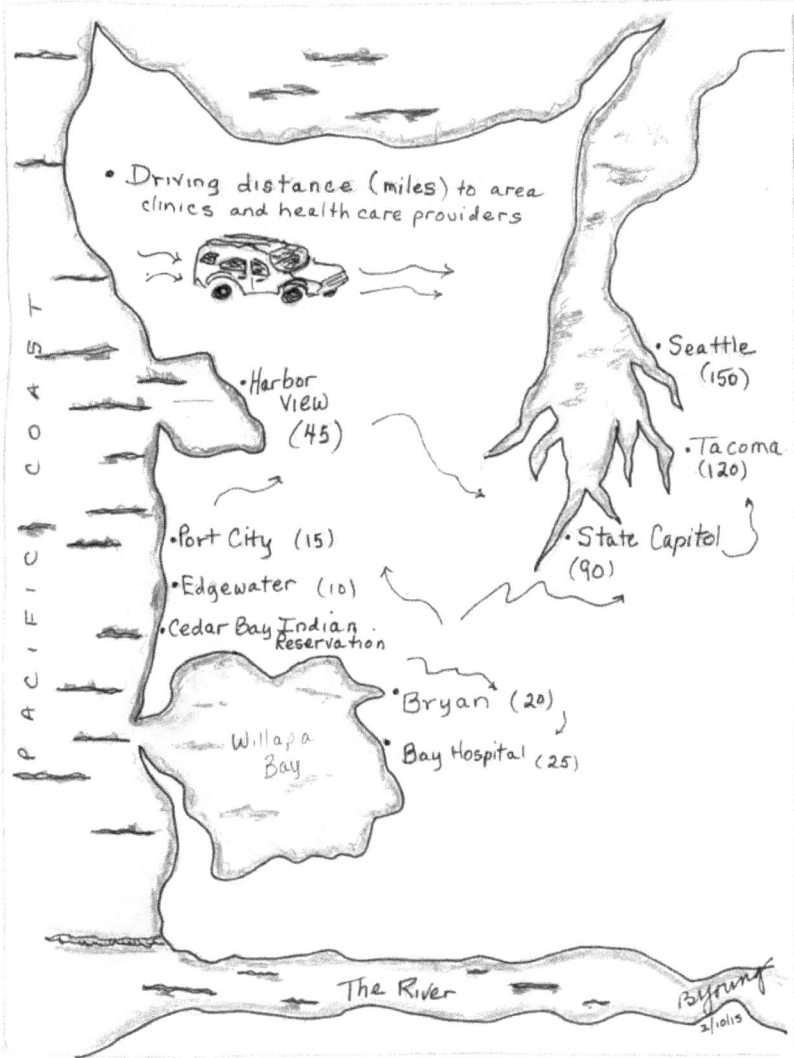

This sketch shows the distance from health care providers and area clinics.

Four Traditional Healers

Shortly after I begin working with the tribe, I leave the reservation to attend the Annual Meeting of the American Public Health Association being held in San Diego. I attend each year because it exposes me to the public health problems and strategies to address them around the globe. An emphasis for me this year is to participate in sessions sponsored by the American Indian, Alaskan Native and Native Hawaiian Caucus.

In the large ballroom, I choose a seat near the aisle and prepare my mind and body to listen. I let go of the conference hustle. I take a deep breath and exhale slowly, concentrating on my breath.

In the front of the ballroom is an elevated platform with four guest speakers. The first speaker approaches the microphone and everyone rises for an opening prayer. By the time we sit down, a calming presence and attentive energy has filled the huge space.

The first presenter is Navajo, a grandfather, leader and spiritual healer. He shares stories of the Southwest, of family, of pottery made with sand, of woven blankets. From him, I receive the gift of story in healing.

The next traditional healer is Apache, also a grandfather, leader, and healer. From him, I receive the gift of humor in healing. We learn to laugh at life. How an Indian leader can find the humor in history and bring life and laughter to a large ballroom is indeed a gift of health.

Traditional healer number three is Alaskan Tlingit, a grandfather with white hair, dressed in seal fur. He gives us stories from the North for our healing. His stories speak of wisdom and the warmth of the family circle.

Traditional healer four is Hawaiian Native, dressed in a brilliant blue, red, and yellow floral short-sleeved shirt. He speaks of his large family on the islands. He gives us the gift of brilliant blooms, time and family.

After the session concludes, I attend the public health nurse lunch meeting. This year, members of the Washington State chapter of Service, Education, and Research in Community Health Nursing will receive the Public Health Nursing Section Lillian Wald Award for collective contributions to the advancement of public health nursing education and practice. I am a member of this organization, and receiving this recognition is an honor. Smiling broadly, we pose for the official group portrait.

After three days of stimulating, thought provoking, and well-delivered presentations, I leave the warmth of San Diego and return to the rain and storms of Willapa Bay.

Humor

Relieves tension. Lightens burdens.

Just when I am beginning to take myself too seriously and focus on the task like a carriage horse in blinders, I find in my mailbox bits of Indian humor. My colleagues and the people of the tribe are telling me that it is time to lighten up. "Chill out," the teens say. "Cool it, Mom," says Susan. Humor brightens the soul. It levels the playing field. I cannot think of a better way to heal than to learn to laugh at myself. The traditional healer in San Diego showed us how. The members of the Cedar Bay Tribe show me how.

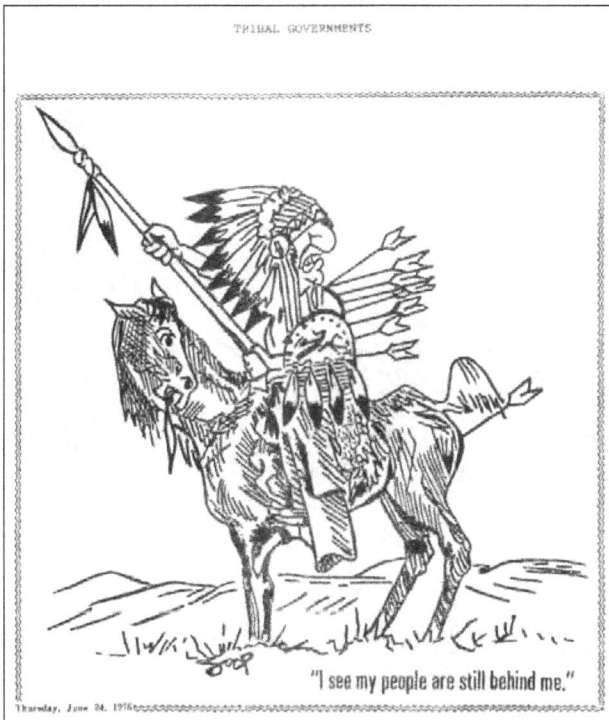

"I see my people are still behind me."

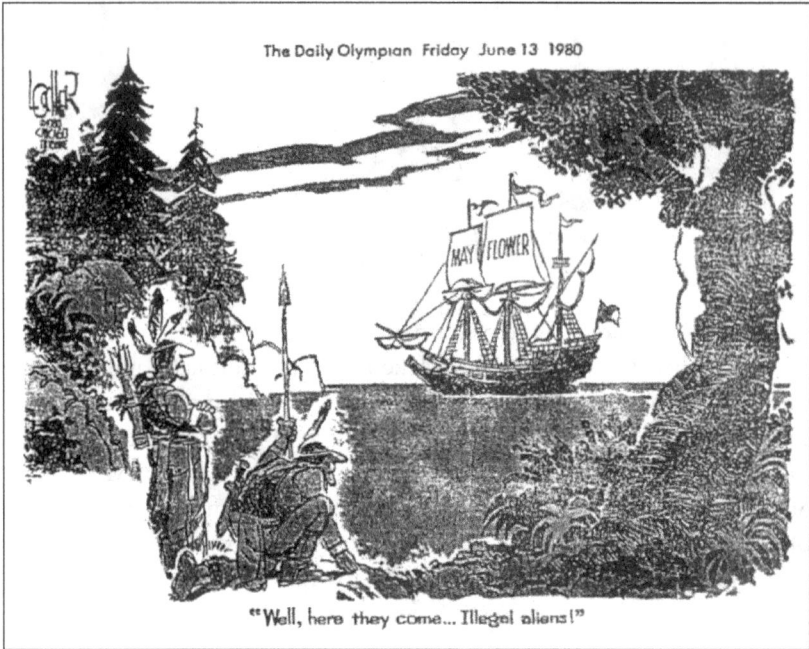

"Well, here they come... Illegal aliens!"

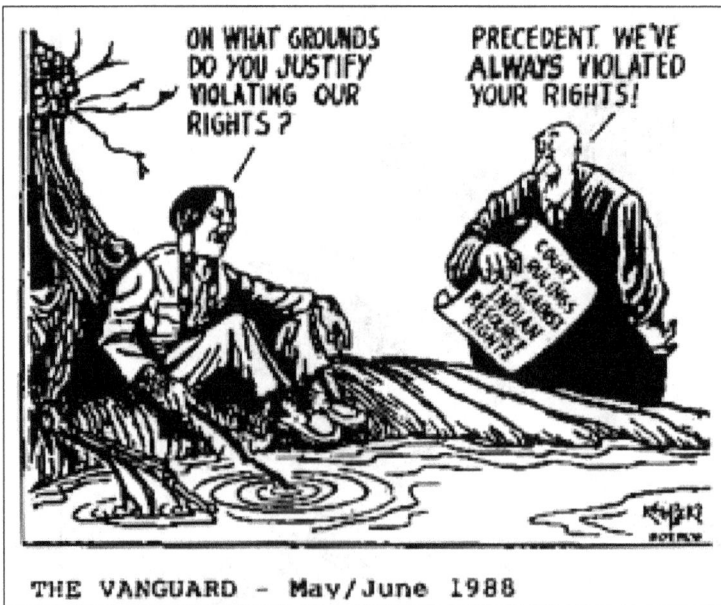

THE VANGUARD - May/June 1988

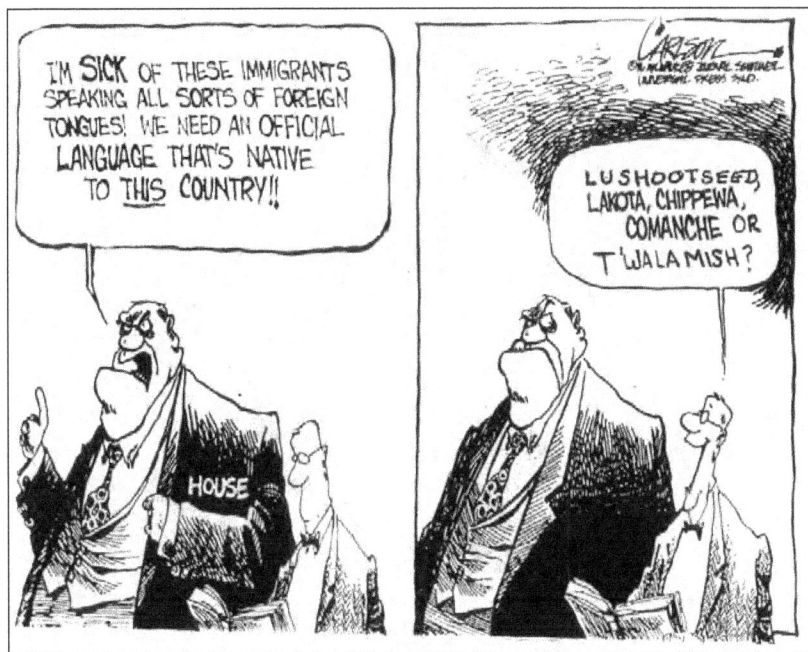

I altered this cartoon by inserting *Lushootseed* and *T'wala mish*, local Native languages of the Lummi Tribe and the Cedar Bay Tribe. Vi Hilbert of the Lummi Tribe made it her life's work to save, describe and teach the *Lushootseed* language, which saved it from extinction.

T'wala mish is the ancient language of the Shaolwater peoples. The tribal education director teaches the language during after-school tutoring sessions with the children of the tribe. This practice reminds me of my high school days when my Jewish friends went to Hebrew school after regular school, to learn the language of their ancestors, and of the Vietnamese refugees who sent their children to school on week-ends to learn their native language.

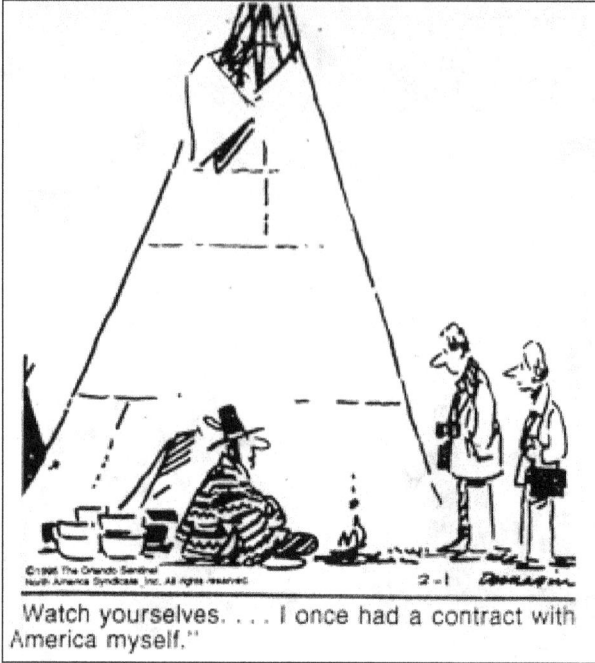

"Watch yourselves. . . . I once had a contract with America myself."

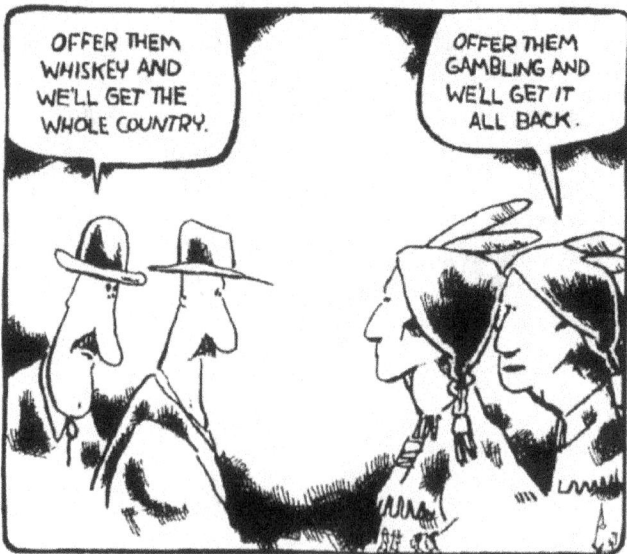

OFFER THEM WHISKEY AND WE'LL GET THE WHOLE COUNTRY.

OFFER THEM GAMBLING AND WE'LL GET IT ALL BACK.

December

Panklich

Time of darkness

Reporter

Sitting across from me in my office at the reservation is a young reporter from the *Chinook Observer*. I want to be sharp in my responses because this article will give an impression to the tribal community and to the entire county why I, a white nurse, had come to work on the reservation.

Reporter: "Why have you come to the reservation?"

"I was hired by the chairman to be the project coordinator of a grant titled Returning to Health: Reducing Sociocultural Barriers to Health Care."

"But why you in particular? Why not a native nurse practitioner or health educator?"

I begin defensively to expound on my experience in the state health department developing the First Steps Prenatal Access program—health care that offered social, nutritional, and public health education visits to ensure healthy pregnancy outcomes. It sounds reasonable. But really—I think to myself, not out loud to the reporter—I am here because I need to learn the lessons myself. I want what I did not know I need—to grieve with the women and the tribe their lost infants, their lost culture, and their lost language. As a representative of the dominant culture, I need to be present, here, at a time of deep grief and to share in that grief. Will there be a future for these people or might they fade away in the eroding tidewaters on the border of their reservation? Will their lessons be lost to us all?

"What are the goals of the grant?" the reporter continues.

"The main goal is to ensure the survival of these people by addressing the ninety-percent infant mortality rate that has already received national attention. The stated objectives of the grant are: form a focus group of women to identify issues, provide the care that is needed, promote quality prenatal health care to native women on the reservation as well as in the county, and develop a model program that can be duplicated." It sounds like a canned recitation; it is easy to quote the objectives right out of the grant, funded from New Jersey and administered from Washington, D.C.

The goals were more simply stated by the chairman: "Empower the women of the tribe to promote their own health care; make the clinic their own. We can teach the world."

"Will anyone listen?" I ask the reporter.

Focus Group

A focus group is a convening of persons to address a specific topic or issue. The following objectives are included in the grant:

- Form a focus group of women to address health concerns.

- Promote health services to the Cedar Bay Indian Nation and to the Native American population of the county.

- Train health staff at the tribal clinic to be culturally sensitive to women's reproductive issues.

- Develop protocol for reproductive health care case management when health care providers are located in communities far from the reservation.

- Write a health care resource guide to be used as a model for other Native American communities.

- *Empower the women* to understand their health care issues and to be health care leaders within their families and the tribal community.

- *Shift ownership* of the tribal clinic from white care providers to the Indian community.

On the reservation and in the tribal clinic, where almost ninety percent of the providers are white, patients do not feel that the clinic is "theirs." The pool of Native American health care providers is small. Recruiting workers to a community reservation clinic at current salary levels and far from medical back-up services is an additional difficulty. How does one provide role models for young Native Americans who might one day staff the clinic?

Eight women, each having suffered a miscarriage or stillbirth, were selected for the focus group. This group will plan the health programs that I will begin to implement.

The initial meeting of the Women's Focus Group is held at 6:00 p.m.

in December on the second floor of the tribal community center. The women form a circle of chairs under the skylight and the meeting begins with a prayer by the community health representative.

> *One Great Spirit and Creator of all things, we ask your guidance and direction on this day. Please open our hearts and ears and minds to the materials and messages delivered to us and shared among us. Give us the wisdom to understand the messages. Give us a sense of our belonging and place in your great plan of life. Let each and every one of us know you have created us as bright, intelligent, loving human beings and that you are always watching us. Remind us of the leadership of our ancestors. Help us to be worthy of the leadership responsibilities you have given us through this meeting. Thank you, Great Spirit and Creator of All Things, for your presence in our lives.*

Following the opening prayer, a member of the group reads the legend of Raven and the creation of the nation. When the story is finished, we proceed to the business portion of our gathering. Large blank sheets of paper are taped to the cedar wall.

The group listens courteously while I state the objectives of the grant, all written by others outside the tribe. They listen to an extensive work plan that has been defined by the funding source in New Jersey. The women sit silently listening as I, with my western-medical-world training wordily and hurriedly ramble on.

Hesitantly at first, the women begin to express their own needs. As they gain confidence, they speak of issues facing their families—nutrition, schooling, jobs, medical care access and lack of transportation. The women do not feel equal to other women sitting in the doctors' waiting rooms. They do not feel that the doctors understand their needs. The sheets of paper fill with words of hurt and sadness. After all the members of the group have spoken, we sit in silence for many minutes.

Then, someone speaks of taking positive action. Others in the group join in. A work plan begins to emerge and as energy becomes focused on the positive, the women's enthusiasm is also documented on the paper: thoughts, ideas, and stories. A mission statement begins to appear. Objectives and goals begin to be formulated. The women put the focus where it needs to be—on their own process of healing, health, and wellness. With the women intensely engaged and their energy focused on work, my mind begins to wander and I remember my early training in

Peace Corps community development and the empowerment teachings of Paulo Friere.

◆ ◆ ◆ ◆ ◆

Thirty years ago, spring was coming to the Vermont mountains when I reported to the School for International Training in Brattleboro. I had been selected to go to the interior of Brazil as a Peace Corps volunteer to work for public health. Ten professors of language immersed the trainees in culture and communication. Federal state department staff trained us in protocols. Educators introduced the philosophy and methods of Paulo Freire, the exiled Brazilian Secretary of Education. His method of community literacy empowered people to participate in planning their own future.

From the 1965 continuing education training book:

> Paulo Freire, Brazilian educator and philosopher, believed that men and women can be empowered to take a critical look at their own awareness and social reality, and can utilize the resulting awareness and sense of self-esteem to transform the social structures that neglect them. Freire believed that everyone is capable of formulating their own thoughts and acting upon them. Men and women, regardless of economic status or educational level, are not "empty vessels" into which information is deposited, but are equipped with the ability to transform their world.

> Freire's methods also promote the awakening of the conscience, which enables one to become aware of the existing social norms and status quo. This awakening leads to the abandonment of an individualistic mentality for a sense of community and a concern for the common good. The student develops a critical, community based mentality through consideration of personal, local problems. The Freire method attempts to abolish apathy; to develop a critical awareness of problems and their causes; and subsequently, to motivate groups of people to become actively involved in solving these problems. He recognizes different levels of consciousness as a link between emotion and the motivation to act; the significance of a curriculum developed by students instead of 'experts,' and the need for development and liberation to originate at the grassroots level. Freire ultimately sought to liberate people, helping them to become critical, creative, free, active and responsible members of society. (Hope and Timmel, 1994) This liberation is achieved in a reciprocal educational exchange between

teacher and students through problem-posing, dialogue, and practical action." (*Building Communities from the Inside Out.* APHA C.E. Institute #2, "The Freire Method: Education and Empowerment for the Underserved")

The Brattleboro training has shaped my work ever since. In the 1960s, I was a new graduate nurse of a big ten school and descendant of Ohio territory pioneers. The sixties were a time of inner-city unrest, John Glenn's ride in space, John Kennedy's oft-repeated quote, *Ask not what your country can do for you, but what you can do for your country*, then his assassination. My own answer to his challenge came in the form of an invitation to train for the Peace Corps and go to Brazil. My husband and I trained for grassroots community development. Paulo Freire was our theoretical tutor, and his book, *Pedogogy of the Oppressed,* became our guidebook.

In 1969, I met Paulo Freire near my home in Cincinnati when he was invited to a Catholic retreat center to lead a seminar on community literacy. Our daughter was four months old. I stayed in the rear of the room so that I could inconspicuously nurse her. As *Senhor* Freire neared the end of his lecture, speaking in English, he asked permission to speak in Portuguese. A translator was present. In the most eloquent Portuguese, he looked at the baby in my arms and spoke of the newborn who nurses from its mother. "*O infante nasceo. Mama. Commences de apreender o mundo pelo os olhos dos paes. Entao, o infante cresceo. O infant commences de rojar-se. Andar. Correr. Cada um e um pedaceo dos desenvolvemento de aprender.* (The infant is born. Nurses. Begins to learn the world through the eyes of the parents. The baby grows. Crawls. Walks. Runs. Each is a step in the development of learning.) Freire's lecture was a lesson in the dynamic process of growth and learning.

◆ ◆ ◆ ◆ ◆

The tribal women of the circle are focused; the words on the wall tell the stories. They have considered the distance to health provider offices, and how their cars are often in disrepair. The women have considered their communications with health care providers, and how widely their cultural interpretations differ. As they consider all of this, my thoughts wander again and I remember a missed communication in a medical consultation between a Latino patient and her Anglo doctor.

Doctor: "Hello. Do you need a translator?"

María: "No, thank you. It's okay." She clearly did not want to impose or incur extra expense.

Doctor: "I'm glad you have come to see me. You have a viral infection. Do you understand?"

María: "Si. Yes. But my throat hurts."

Doctor: "I know; it is very red. Drink lots of fluids. Take Tylenol every four hours and get lots of rest. Do you understand?"

María: "Si, doctor. Gracias."

Doctor: (thinking to himself) I wonder if she understood what I said.

María's son: "Mom, can we go now? I am hungry. What did the doctor say? What is wrong?"

María:"He told me to rest. Ha! With four kids? We waited for two hours. And the doctor didn't give me a shot. All I got was a piece of paper in English, and I can't read what it says."

Each was operating within their own cultural norms and perceptions; neither knew how to bridge the barriers to their misunderstanding.

❖ ❖ ❖ ❖ ❖

I remember another story of miscommunication that resulted in the tragic death of twin infants. It was at the health care clinic in Brazil. A mother of newborn twins who the *visitadora* (the equivalent of a U.S. visiting home health care aide) and I had previously visited in her home had not returned to the health clinic for her infants' six-week checkup. We were making another home visit to find out why. The mother told us the babies died. "Diarrhea," she says. I am stunned. Why did she not return to get help?

❖ ❖ ❖ ❖ ❖

Back at the reservation, fresh paper is added to our charts. "What do you want this picture to look like in three years?" I ask. The women of the circle planning group consider and reply:

"I want to be treated fairly and with respect."

"I want the provider to be a woman who understands me."

"I want to wait for my visit with the provider only a reasonable amount of time."

"I want to feel better."

The meeting comes to a close. We stand in a circle while the community health worker leads us in a closing prayer. The women leave for their homes and families. I move the sheets from the cedar panels to the bare walls of my office. The words are beacons in the lighthouse of a dark night.

The World Health Organization states:

> Health is a state of complete physical, mental and social well-being, and not merely the absence of disease or infirmity. The human factor is what is important in determining health and well-being. ... Poverty lies behind the ills of most people. ... Hunger in the world is not primarily due to population growth or shortage of land and resources, rather, it results from unfair distribution of land, resources, and decision-making power. ... Health depends less on technical than on social factors. The healthy person, family, community or nation is one that is relatively self-reliant—one that can relate to others in a helpful, friendly way, as an equal. Health means self-reliance. The health worker's primary job is to help people gain greater control over their health and their lives.

The next week the women gather around the table under the skylight. They begin with prayer and the reading of an Indian legend. The community health worker has a box of beads, string and needles. She explains the meaning of the colors. Brilliant blue is for spirituality. Amber is of the earth. White is for purity. Green is growth. Black is reflection. Red is the blood of life. Yellow is the sun. Crystal is for clarity. The women select beads. They give themselves permission to be creative. It never occurred to me to use the colors, the art, the soothing touch of beads, and the act of creating patterns as an expression of working through grant objectives. I considered this a frivolous activity, one to participate in only when the "real" work was done. I am learning that the real work begins as we center ourselves with this activity. The women laugh and tell stories and discuss their work as they create. They prioritize work and plan activities, guided by the colors of the beads.

Priority One: Open a women's clinic. Promote the clinic to the women of the tribal community and Native American women in the surrounding county.

Priority Two: Understand the relationship of diabetes to health and daily living.

Priority Three: Identify personal health behaviors relating to alcohol, tobacco and drugs, and with this increased knowledge become empowered to implement change.

The necklaces the women make become gifts. Four are selected to be given to the grant evaluation team, scheduled to visit the reservation soon.

For a return to health, there must be balance. Many trained in western medicine are now recognizing how important it is to offer patients of various ethnicities alternatives for healing. Others are studying alternative and complementary medicine to incorporate these approaches into their own practices. Healing seems to take place when we speak the language and understand the culture.

I return again to the concept of the medicine wheel and its four directions. The east represents the beginning, the sun rising, the birth, the seedling, the child; south—warmth, growth, development, adolescence; west—maturity, reflection, pause, darkness, depth; and north—elder, white hairs and wisdom, cold and ice. Life is a circle from birth to elder to rebirth and on around the circle. The community health worker says that the medicine wheel has been a part of the culture for thousands of years, an integral part of their lives. I am new to this ancient wisdom. I am an outsider who wants to be inside the circle. I want to explore its depth and meaning. If I am the center of my own healing circle, then I must heal my mental, spiritual, emotional, and physical ailments to gain balance and harmony in health.

◆ ◆ ◆ ◆ ◆

My daughter Susan has been studying Celtic mythology as part of the Society of Creative Anachronism, a black-clad group she recently joined at the nearby college. She shows me a picture from a book she is reading. The caption reads, "The Gundestrup cauldron is a silver-plated copper bowl discovered in 1891 in a peat bog at Gundestrup in Denmark and is believed to have belonged to the first or second century B.C." The bowl is highly decorated. The relief on the side of the caldron is the deity Taranis, a healer. His hands are raised. His symbol is the wheel.

Susan shares what she's learned about the symbolism of the Celtic cross and the four directions. East is air; south, fire; west, water; and north, ice. I visualize the four directions with colors. They would be: east, yellow; south, red; west, black; north, white. Roy Wilson, Cowlitz Indian Chairman and Methodist minister, compares the Four Directions with the Four Gospels of Christianity. He is native. I am non-native, but through our ancient heritages, we are connected. Through our religious ceremonies and beliefs, we are connected.

◆ ◆ ◆ ◆ ◆

The group continues to meet, plan and become stronger in their commitment to implement change. However, the women's group draws criticism from the grant funding source. The group and its actions are not considered by the academic and funding communities to be a legitimate "focus group." A true focus group is defined in the academic literature as a group called together for a short period to define an area of study. Because of this narrow definition, and the silly criticism that they are not an official focus group, the women agree to be called "Women's Planning Group." In defense of their work and in defiance of a definition from someone "off reservation" telling them who they are and are not, the women retreat to their *T'walamish* vocabulary list to search for the native words for "focus group." They know very well that they have the answers to the questions being asked from the outside funding source. Their group is the focus.

Tun n. T wal'mes. T mt's. Xa c. Tum. Yul'w n. Cic . T c. Mi a Latam. It doesn't work. A direct translation from *T'walamish* to English isn't possible. History, customs, and culture have been passed down by oral tradition and sometimes lost through disease and the death of the storytellers. The women are left with the title "Women's Planning Group," which proves acceptable to the grant funding source. They empowered themselves to define the focus of their work. The name does not matter. The Women's Planning Group is in practice and in reality, a focus group. They develop rules.

Rules for the Women's Planning Group to feel safe:

- *Share time equally.* Each member takes a turn speaking. This should be flexible so that if someone has a great deal to say, they should be able to do so. The time needs of the other people in the group should also be taken into account; therefore, the group should have some idea of how much time is available for each member.

- *Protect confidentiality.* No personal information about any group member should be discussed outside the group. A general observation, without names and details, can be used for processing purposes.

- *Listen to each person attentively without interrupting.* Each person has an important experience to relate that should not be judged or challenged. Feelings are valid; no one is told how to feel.

- *Speak about your personal experiences.* People learn from personal experiences.

- *Strive for complete honesty.* This need not conflict with protecting the feelings of others.

- *Avoid side remarks.* Share all remarks with the group. Comments, questions and opinions are of interest to all members.

Doodling

James Thurber, of Walter Mitty fame, doodled on the restroom wall in the Scandia restaurant in Hollywood. I know this because I have seen the doodles. Now, I am doodling page after page trying to figure out a connection between the medicine wheel and the state's Public Health Improvement Plan.

The Public Health Improvement Plan incorporates program planning, implementation, and evaluation—from programs addressing communicable disease and environmental health to personal injury and safety. The project grant that supports my work at the reservation states its mission in the title, *Opening Doors: Reducing Sociocultural Barriers to Health Care*. In Celtic culture, my brother tells me, there is a body of knowledge relating to health and wellness that derives from the ancient Druid healers.

Each of our cultures has its own history of medical practice. In the native cultures of the Pacific Northwest, the wisdom and medicine for health and healing was passed down through oral storytelling, dance and sweat lodge. When these cultures were decimated, the tribes lost their connection to medicine and to their vital healing ceremonies.

Does culture and ancient knowledge intersect with today's dominant health care system? Does the dominant culture even recognize the possibilities of health and healing that exist within ancient healing traditions?

More doodling. The book *The Power of Ten* begins at the scale of the whole universe, then moves slowly down to the parts of an atom. Beginning with LARGE and moving to small stimulates my thinking. I consider the women of the tribe working to heal their loss and grief, and I begin to see how healing energy from the whole universe flows to these individual lives.

Healing energy flows from the universe to the smallest particle.

Healing energy flows from the universe to each tribal member, and then in reverse, from each tribal member back to the universe. I can apply this concept to the dominant culture health care systems.

Policy flows from Washington, D.C. and affects individual members of the women's group.

When the women decide that they are ready to share their stories so that others might heal from them, this healing energy flows back, and can serve the system as a whole—if the dominant culture is prepared to receive and respect it.

We are all truly interconnected and can share in the healing process.

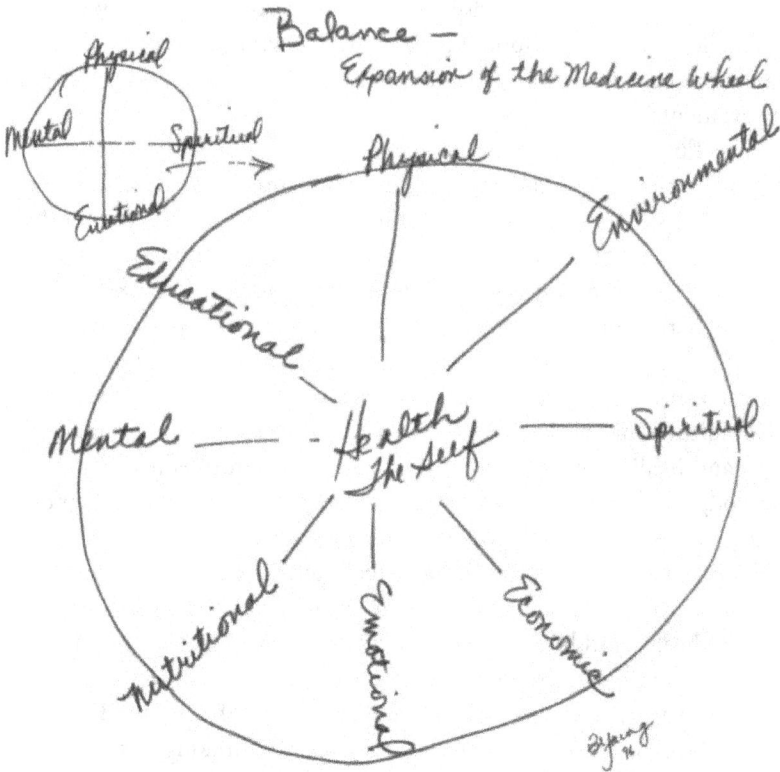

After talking with the chairman, I draw additional spokes on a medicine wheel balancing physical, mental, emotional and spiritual health. The additions are educational, environmental, nutritional, and economic.

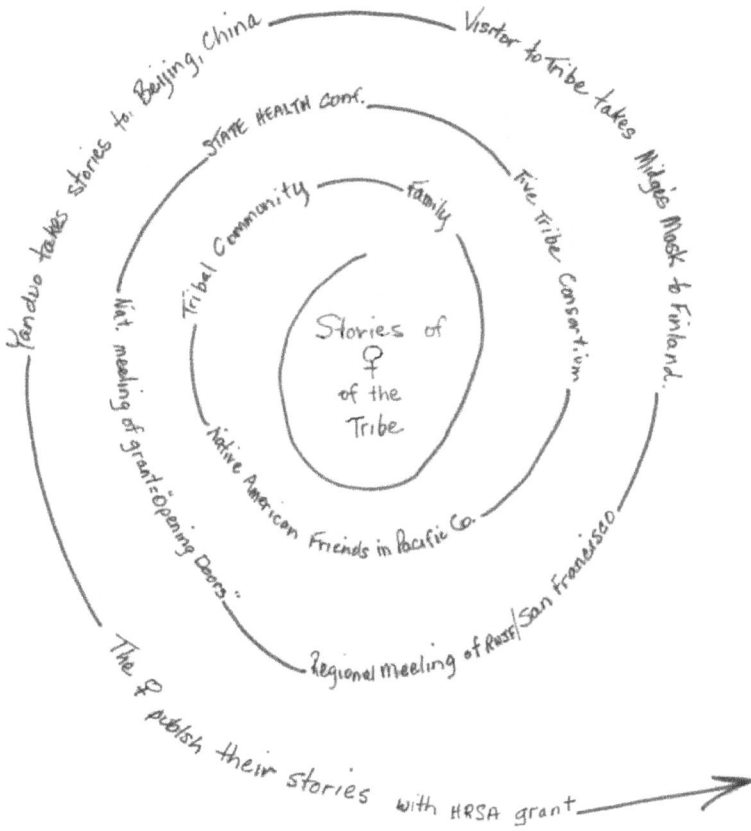

The women of the tribe make plaster of Paris masks to express their life stories as they mourn lost infants. They write their stories to share with others and contribute to a book. Their sharing spirals outward to their families, then the tribal community, the county and the world. The stories are specifically carried to Finland and to China via visitors to the tribal community.

January

Panpamas

Time of cold

Tribal Women's Health

The mammogram mobile unit arrives at the reservation for its scheduled visit. Appointment slots are filled. An elder, She-Who-Knows, is first—her breasts squashed against hard plastic plates on the stand-up X-ray. She complains of a pain in one of her breasts. The X-ray results come back within the week and she is to report to the clinic in Bryan for a biopsy. After waiting again for her biopsy results, She-Who-Knows is told to report for another test to Capital Medical Center in Olympia, eighty-two miles from the reservation. As she enters the cancer clinic, she recognizes a large art display, *Traditional Healing Medicines*, built by her friend—a nurse practitioner and shaman. The art features a medicine bag, tobacco leaves, abalone shell, feathers and sweet grass. She feels the healing energy of the display and is encouraged.

She-Who-Knows undergoes more tests and waits to hear. This time the explanation comes in the form of a pen sketch on paper that describes the location of the cancer and how the surgical removal of the breast starting at the outer quadrant and moving toward the nipple can remove the cancer and save her life. She is scheduled for a right radical mastectomy.

Before the surgery, in a hospital far from home, family and friends gather at her bedside, a medicine bag close by. Prayers are given. It is time for grief and loss. Humor is also a part of the good medicine, and the group tells stories, laughs and enjoys life.

Following surgery, She-Who-Knows begins a series of chemotherapy treatments resulting in fatigue and loss of hair. Throughout this time of therapy and healing, she remains courageous. Months after the surgery, there is no stronger advocate for the women's health program than She-Who-Knows. She receives great respect, not only for her courage in facing her diagnosis, but for her push to have all tribal women receive access to services for early detection of breast and cervical cancer. It is an intense and important start to the year.

Reflections

It is time for me to pause and think of how all this relates to my own life. I take a deep breath. I am "sitting" a bayside home while the owner winters in the Southwest and I invite my sister and her friend Micki to join me. They, too, could use some time by the bay to relax and reflect.

Before the sun comes up, I awaken. I get up, light the oil lamp and place it on the table by the large bay window. I write as the sunlight wakes up the sleeping village. The day is grey, as it should be in January in the Pacific Northwest. The wings of the blue jay weather vane turn softly. The children's empty swing in the backyard, hanging from a lone fir, gently sways ever so slightly. I am alone with my thoughts.

Friends—Lois from Cincinnati and Caroline from Houston—called me this past weekend. Was I okay? What was I doing now? Neither had received my annual Christmas letter, because this year I didn't send one.

"Did you get your chores done?" My sister asks me. She does not know that I, like the author Leoni in his story *Frederick the Mouse*, am allowing others to gather the grain for winter while I am busy collecting stories for the dark months ahead.

Neighbor Einor, who recited his poem *Winds of the Willapa* in soft lamp light after a dinner of poached fresh salmon, has just been diagnosed with prostate cancer. Although my assignment here at the reservation is focused on women's health, I am reminded of the prevalence of cancer in both women and men.

Rains blow sideways at the shoal waters. I see it in the street light. I am getting wet standing under the roofed entrance of the community center.

Captain Phil studies the tide tables. He discusses the preparation and packs food, water, and warm jackets. He gasses the boat and readies for departure to Long Island and the Trail of the Ancient Cedars.

Micki is saying something that is relevant to my writing and the reasons for low birth weight babies. She is talking about her daughter's birth and her grandmother and.... My mind stops and focuses on what she is telling me. Her grandmother was one-quarter Indian, from the Iowa tribe in the area of southern Minnesota. Micki's daughter was born in 1966, with a blue spot the size of a Kennedy half dollar at the base of her spine. Micki had been frightened. Her baby was born prematurely and weighed three pounds, two ounces. Had someone dropped her baby, leaving a bruise? The doctor relieved her fears. "It is genetic, an inherited trait of those of Mediterranean, Italian, Greek, and Native American descent." The spot fades after a few months." As to the question of premature birth, Micki explains that the hospital in Racine, Wisconsin, is prepared and even anticipates low birth weight and premature babies because research shows that in this area, premature births are related to the barometric pressure and the geography of Lake Michigan.

Three women of the tribal community go to the other Washington to tell their stories of tribal loss. They display eleven tribal masks. Without words, the masks express the stories of loss, grief and courage. A young Latino woman from an inner-city Chicago clinic approaches the women, and embraces them with understanding.

In a communications workshop in San Francisco, statements are written on a flip chart. I lead the discussion of the tribe's need to communicate their losses. "Their tragedy resonates with us all. Their survival is the survival of us all." As the discussion becomes more lively and addresses communication across cultural barriers, I begin to think that maybe there *is* a way to communicate the tribe's loss. Perhaps the east coast experts *can* understand the connection between this small tribe and the wellbeing of all people.

I imagine a letter written to the tribal chairman. "Dear Chairman, has the health of the women improved since the emergency was declared? The tribe's survival and prosperity is vital to us all. Everywhere I go, New York City, Washington, D.C., San Francisco, Albuquerque and Chicago, people ask me, "What is the cause of infant mortality?" An invisible link connects all people to the tribe and to one another. We are connected—you and I. You are called to lead; I, to write. The Great Spirit has given tasks for us both. It is survival—your people, my people and peoples everywhere. We are all connected."

My nurse friend Joyce brought me a round gold pin from a nursing meeting in California, showing children holding hands around the world. The pin brings me joy.

Basket Class

I place the coiled basket I am working on under the kitchen faucet and let it collect a small pool of water. Will it be watertight like the tiny stitched baskets of the ancient Chinook? Or will it resemble the baskets that were used to gather berries? I pour out the water, afraid to test it further. Loose ends of sweet grass signify I need to continue the arduous work. Stitch over stitch. Hour after hour. I shift my bifocals to the top of my head so that I can see how close together I have stitched the raffia over the sweet grass. One tribal member gave me sweet grass she harvested. Another gave me colored raffia. The raffia comes from Southeast Asia and was purchased from a craft store. In the Pacific Northwest the ancestral Indian women gathered raffia discarded from trade boats in the ports near Seattle. Used for packing, the raffia was tossed overboard and eventually washed ashore.

The women of the Monday evening basket class form a circle with their chairs and pull out their sweet grass, cattails, raffia, needles and baskets in different stages of completion. "You are making good progress," the elder tells me. I smile. I have been working on this basket for two winters. "Your design is nice. Soon you will be starting the lid." I do not reply. The project has taken every ounce of my patience and I thought I would not make the lid, although it is customary to do so for Chinook baskets.

"Mine wants to be an open basket," I respond.

"No, it doesn't. The lid will make your basket complete."

"It will teach you discipline," another adds.

"You need it," still another of the circle says. Women around the circle chuckle and enjoy the humor. Remaining silent this time, I contemplate the lid and continue the stitching, pushing the raffia needle over the sweet grass, stitch by stitch, coil over coil, row over row.

One of the women begins to tell a story. The others listen as they stitch. This is a circle of women who work to revive ancient basket weaving skills. In the past, baskets were used in trade—in addition to being functional tools. The beauty and refinement of the Chinook baskets are known throughout the region, up and down the Pacific coast and inland to the waterways that empty into the Columbia.

The elder tells of the basket museum that once existed on the reservation, containing hundreds of baskets made by tribal artists. She shares pictures, of shelves of baskets for every function of gathering and cooking. "There are none left on the reservation," the Elder says. "They were all sold at auction because the owner wanted the money and did not realize the baskets' true value to the tribe. The baskets are probably all over the Pacific Northwest but not in Indian homes."

I am reminded of what the chairman said when I asked him to explain the reason for the current emphasis upon building a casino, which seems to me in direct conflict with the isolated beauty and peacefulness of the reservation lands. He said, "We have lost our baskets. If we could have an income, we could buy back our baskets. We could touch our culture and hold onto our past."

The elder allows me to hold the one remaining family basket she keeps at home. The design of contrasting natural and black provides a stair step effect that goes from bottom to top and back to bottom. It is strikingly simple yet remarkably strong. I think of the women, grandparents and great grandparents of the women of the circle who came together in similar circles to weave, to tell of family problems, and to gain support from the other women in the circle. My needle sews the raffia over the sweet grass, stitch over stitch.

One woman in the circle speaks of the difficulty of communicating with her teen-age son. We sit in silence, weaving, and let her pain move around the circle; all absorbing a piece of it, grieving with the mother who had spoken. It doesn't matter whether we are Chinook, Celtic or Chinese. The women of the circle understand and share in the grief.

The elder speaks next. "My mother went to the boarding school, Chamagwa. She had to work in the kitchen and learn domestic skills. Mom had a very mean supervisor who yelled at her. Nothing Mom did was ever right. Finally, one day, my mother had enough of the criticism. She picked up a large bag of flour, dumped it over the head of the supervisor and walked out of the kitchen. Mother was never reprimanded. I guess the supervisor knew she deserved the dumping." There are chuckles around the circle.

Another tells of an injured crow she is nursing in her house. In black raffia, a crow is woven into the woman's basket as part of the family's story.

Two hours of basket class pass quickly. We collect our weaving materials and say good night. On nights like these, power outages on the bay are frequent. Our meeting space will soon be occupied by another group. The tribal center opens its doors to the local Alcoholics Anonymous chapter. Non-native members come from the surrounding community and are joined by tribal residents. They, too, work methodically, step by step. AA group members help other members, in a sense, to put on a lid—completing their own project which could be called "recovery for sobriety."

As I head up the dark coast toward home, I think of my own ancestors and how the women gathered on winter evenings to discuss family concerns and gain support and understanding from the seniors. On those severe Ohio winter days when the ground was covered in deep snow, the women gathered in the attic of the valley farmhouse. There they circled around a quilt frame and pieced together scraps from worn dresses. They, too, sewed their stories of grief, humor and healing.

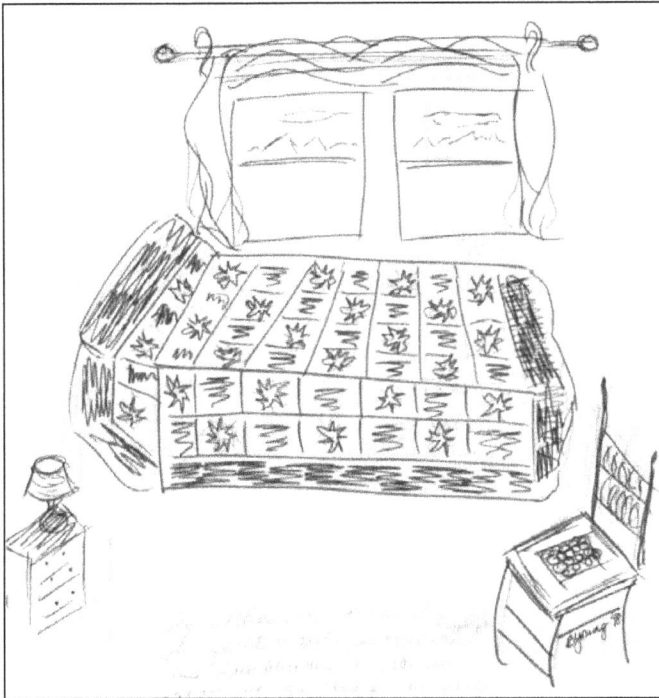

This quilt has an eight-point star pattern with alternating squares of royal blue fabric with tiny white stars. My mother's grandmother quilted it and gave it to my mother on the occasion of her birth, September 5, 1903 in Columbus, Ohio. The quilt was made on the old frame in the attic of the farmhouse in the Pee Pee Valley of Pike County in southern Ohio.

February

Panlaleah-kilech

Time of beach willow

Diabetes Class

The Seattle Post-Intelligencer runs an article indicating that diabetes might be one of the culprits in high infant mortality. The Women's Planning Group wants to check this out. Priority number one is to establish the women's health clinic. Priority number two is to learn more about diabetes: a class is planned.

Invitations and notices go out to those in the clinic service area. The local radio station and newspapers carry public service announcements. The clinic staff promotes the class throughout the reservation. Jan Norman, national vice-president of the Diabetes Education Association, agrees to teach the class.

A few people come from as far as Bay City—forty-five miles away. As class participants enter the meeting room, clinic staff check their blood sugar levels with a "finger stick." A finger is pricked for a drop of blood that is examined by the technician. The results of the finger sticks are reported to the participants shortly after the meeting starts. Jan asks the participants why they have come to a diabetes class.

"My family has this disease, and I wonder how I might avoid getting it."

"I want to learn if it played a role in my difficult pregnancy."

"My grandmother suffered with diabetes. I want to learn more about it."

"I have diabetes and want to learn what I can do," says the chairman, who is sitting in the back of the room.

Jan speaks to the tribal leader. "If you wish to slip out for some crackers and then return, that would be okay. Your blood sugar is low today."

"It is difficult," some say, "to maintain a healthy diet on commodity foods which are delivered to the reservation." Others in the class speak of inadequate access to medical supervision and clear explanations from their doctors about the disease. There seems to be a general acceptance of the statistics that show a high incidence of diabetes in Native Americans compared to the general population. The class continues by considering the need to balance a good diet with exercise and regular medical supervision. After an informative and interactive discussion, the class breaks for a diabetic sensitive lunch.

The buffet looks inviting and turns out, to the surprise of all, to be quite tasty. "Can you imagine?" "This is good!"

A welcoming bowl in the chairman's office now no longer contains candy, but fruit. The chairman now takes his work break by walking around the neighborhood. The teacher and the nurse provide information, but it is the tribal leader who is the role model for healthy change.

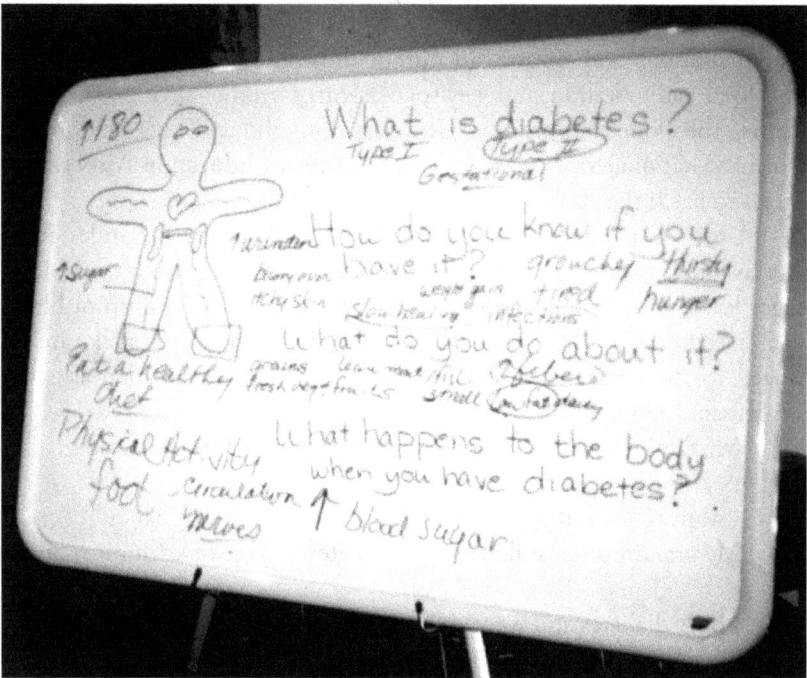

Women's Healing Circle

According to my Cedar Bay friends, word will be circulated by "moccasin telegraph." "Meet in two days in the social hall of the Catholic Church where LeAnn is a member. Bring a bead and a potluck dish." It will be a women's healing circle for LeAnn.

My friend Joyce, who is LeAnn's nursing professor at Seattle University, picks me up for the drive to the church. LeAnn is a public health nurse studying for her master's in nursing and has recently been diagnosed with cancer. Fearing a difficult prognosis, family and friends are coming together to form a healing circle around her.

Women begin to arrive and place various dishes on a long receiving table. Forty of us—native and non-native friends, relatives, colleagues from work, and fellow nursing students come. The gathering begins by offering thanks for the creatures large and small, for the day that brings us together, for LeAnn and her work, and for the food. We feast. After eating, we prepare the circle. One woman offers holy water from a monastery in Nepal. We sprinkle water on our hands as a symbol of washing in prayerful preparation. Another woman, using a feather fan, smudges us by wafting sage smoke burning in an abalone shell. These are rituals of cleansing— blowing away illness, disease, and evil spirits—before we enter the circle. We are to take into the circle only good and clean spirits.

We draw our chairs into a tight circle. Five women walk into the center beating drums; the rhythm calls us to focus. After a few moments of drumming one of the women beckons me into the inner drum circle. She hands me her drum. I listen, and then begin to beat in the same rhythm. My anxiety of trying something new gives way to a peaceful centering. The drums gradually become less intense and slow to a whisper. Focus turns to LeAnn. Members of the circle listen as LeAnn speaks of her illness, the diagnosis and what she is going to do for treatment. "I am going to try experimental drug therapy, and am quite hopeful that this therapy will make a difference. The research is promising." LeAnn is giving herself, and us, hope. A cousin on the other side of the circle tries hard to stifle sobs. LeAnn says that our circle of healing is being duplicated on the Pine Ridge Reservation in the American heartland, where her mother's Lakota Sioux tribe lives. Healing energy will be drawn from both gatherings and strengthen the healing process.

We introduce ourselves around the circle and explain how we know and love LeAnn. Next, a long string is passed. Each woman places a bead on the string. One bead is from Thailand, another is from a mother's wedding necklace. One was worn in a 1960's protest march. Buttons from favorite dresses are added to the string. After the string passes around the circle, a beautiful, eclectic necklace emerges. LeAnn places it around her neck. Each bead and button fits into the whole, and the whole is as it should be, perfect.

A large leather drawstring medicine bag now passes around the circle. Into the bag each woman places good medicine: a poem, a thought or other special item. A few blow healing wishes into the bag. I place three small stones that I had previously gathered from Long Island. LeAnn receives the medicine bag, clutches it closely and says, "Thank you for your energy and for your good medicine." The women close the circle with prayers of thanksgiving and celebration of life.

◆ ◆ ◆ ◆ ◆

I reflect on being in nursing school over thirty years ago, when most of our education focused on physical healing and little on mental health healing. In my first job after graduation—working on the surgical floor of a Seventh Day Adventist hospital, I began to connect with the importance of spiritual healing. I was team-leader on the evening shift and many of the team members had been missionaries in various parts of the world. Evening shift followed a day's busy surgery schedule. When a patient was ready for sleep, the assigned team member asked if they wished a prayer or meditation for their healing. The patient often said, "Yes." I found this to be a comforting time for patient and staff. Prayer brought balance and harmony to the healing process.

My tribal friends taught me to think of the medicine wheel to achieve harmony and balance. The Women's Healing Circle brought spirituality to the healing process for LeAnn. The combined energy of forty spirited women in a social hall would assist in bringing the harmony and balance of the Medicine Wheel for her healing journey.

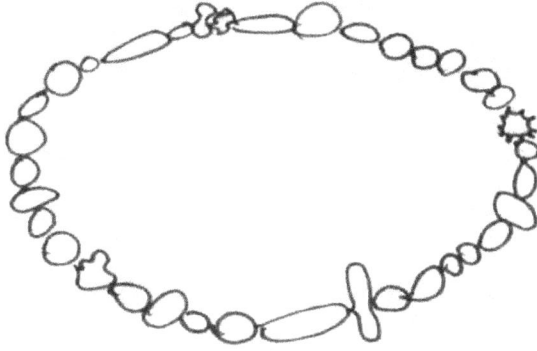

Each bead and button gave its own beauty and energy to the whole.

Talking Circle

"What goes around, comes around," says my friend. She is describing a circle. My students know to re-arrange the chairs in a circle when they come to class. We see and hear each other better. "We learn so much in a circle," they say.

I am invited to lecture at a Tuesday morning family and community health nursing class on the University of Washington Bothell campus eighty miles north of my home. It is the last class before the students receive their Bachelor of Nursing degrees. Class begins at 8:30 and ends at noon. To avoid some of the morning commute, I leave after work on Monday and stay overnight.

When I arrive for class early Tuesday morning to set up, students assist in displaying baskets and hanging pictures of masks from my favorite "Spirit Mask" and "Gathering" calendars. I begin with a reading from Ann Wilson Schaef's book *Native Wisdom for White Minds*, then I tell of my journey as a public health nurse with a small tribe that wants to survive. I share the healing lessons I have learned from the women and men and also the expressive art of the children.

When the students return from break, we arrange the chairs in a circle. Some sit on the floor. The circle is somewhat oblong but still provides the opportunity for all fifty students to face into the center. Lights are dimmed. I read another excerpt from Schaef's book. Rules of the talking circle are reviewed. A talking stick is passed around the circle and the person holding it speaks or shares. Others listen. What is discussed or shared in the circle remains within the circle. Comments made in circle are supportive, positive and reflective, not negative, critical or hurtful. When someone does not wish to speak, they may pass the stick to the next person in the circle.

The talking stick I use came from a walk I had taken on the beach north of Disappointment Point near the mouth of the Columbia River. It is a sturdy, bleached piece of driftwood that has been gnawed on each end. Perhaps it broke loose from a beaver lodge up stream. I pass the stick to the left, noticing that the room is respectfully quiet. My role as facilitator is now to fade into the shadow of the circle. The stick passes around the circle for the first round, each student making a comment if they wish. On the second round the stick is placed on a table in the center of the circle. Each student places a gift on the table—a pen, poems, candy bars, or other objects of importance that helped them through the nursing program. On the third round students select an object that speaks to them. After the discussion, the circle happily adjourns for a potluck lunch celebrating course completion and the graduation ceremony to come.

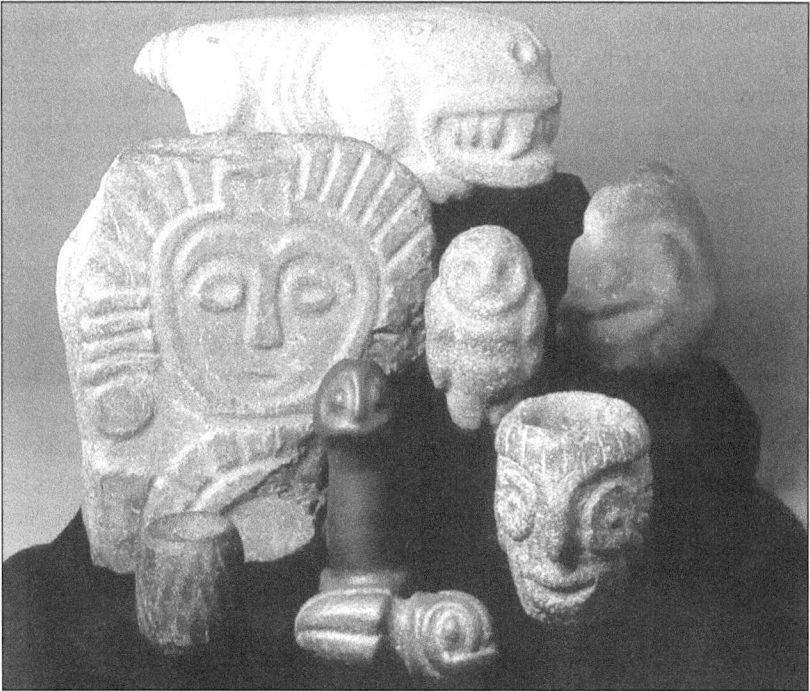

"The Gathering" by Jerry Taylor from a postcard at the Maryhill Museum. These stone sculptures came from ancient Native American cultures along the Columbia River. They represent the beauty of diversity, strength and hope found in any group.

March

Panjans

Time of the sprouts

Health Conference

Winter has passed. Spring has come. It is a time of planting new seeds. On the Christian calendar, it is Easter, the resurrection of life over death. On the Medicine Wheel, it is the east, the rising sun, a new day and a new season. The women of the Planning Group have identified priority three: receive training to understand health care issues among Native American Peoples. It is a time for planting new seeds and learning.

Eight women of the tribal community express the desire to participate in a Native American conference, *Wellness and Women*, to be held in Portland, Oregon. Family and work responsibilities in addition to financial constraints eliminate half that number. Four women and I ride in the tribal education van to Portland where approximately five hundred Native women from all over the country are gathering. Our small group is swept up in the energy.

We select these conference sessions to attend:

- HIV/AIDS
- Sexually Transmitted Diseases
- Traditional Healing Ceremony
- Storytelling for Emotional Healing
- Alcohol and Substance Abuse
- Smoking
- Community Health Representative Program in Rural Alaska
- Inner and Outer Beauty
- Drumming
- Dancing
- Healing from Grief and Loss
- Massage Therapy

- Touch Therapy
- Computer Technology in Health Promotion
- Potlatch

We begin our first conference day at 6:30 a.m. with stretching and then a brisk walk along the banks of the Columbia River. Our leader is heavy set, muscular and energetic and will not let her followers lag behind. A few men among forty women power-walk the distance, gripping the crest at the edge of the river and skirting riverside condominiums. In an hour, we cover about four miles, talking all the way. For the rest of the day, we attend health sessions.

Smoking Health Session

It is important to teach the adverse effects of smoking before and during pregnancy. It is advised to avoid smoking after delivery as well—since newborns, infants, children and others confined to the home cannot excuse themselves from second-hand smoke. Tobacco is a sacred plant to Native Americans, used for ceremony and prayer and to sanctify a sacred space. Today, tobacco is a salable product in every culture. Two flyers distributed in the smoking session show some tobacco-related statistics, women and tobacco use, and the origin of tobacco:

Tobacco-Related Statistics:
- Indian Health Service (IHS) statistics show two out of five deaths of Indians are related to smoking.
- Portland Area IHS lists diseases of the heart as a leading cause of all deaths. Smoking is the most preventable factor in heart disease.
- 90% of lung cancers are smoking related.
- Across all IHS areas, lung cancer is the leading cause of death.
- Smokers are twice as likely to die from lung cancer as nonsmokers.
- Smoking is directly responsible for 433,000 deaths yearly.
- American Indians and Alaskan Natives have the highest rates of tobacco use among ethnic groups.
- A 1989 study in Oregon, Washington and Idaho reported 46% of Indian men and 54% of Indian women smoke as compared to the United States average of 25% for each. 43.5% of adolescents use smokeless tobacco.

- 54% of American Indian women in the Northwest smoke.

- Smoking increases the risk of breast and cervical cancer.

- In Oregon, 33% of American Indian women smoke during pregnancy. This is the highest rate of any ethnic group.

- In Washington, American Indians have the highest infant mortality and sudden infant death rates. High smoking rates are noted on birth and death certificates.

- Female smokers have more miscarriages, stillbirths, premature births, and low birth weight babies.

- American Indian teenage girls have the highest rates of chewing tobacco use.

In 1992, the National Cancer Institute funded a project that compiled stories and facts about traditional Native American tobacco usage. The project, "Reducing Cancer Risks Among Native American Youth in the Northeast," was sponsored by the Columbia University School of Social Work. Although these stories come from the tribes of the eastern United States, they are shared by other Indian nations. They tell of attitudes as well as traditions in the use of tobacco.

Origin of Tobacco (Nipmucks)
By Little Turtle, Nipmuck Tribe, Dudley Band
From: Concord Museum, Concord, MA, c. 1988

> Long ago, there was a wise and peace-loving elder who traveled from tribe to tribe encouraging cooperation and friendship between all nations. He was a spokesman for the cause of good will and his mission was to promote unity among all beings.
>
> At a very great age the elder called a meeting of other elders and representatives from the many clans, tribes, and nations which he had visited and taught. He told them that his work was ending and he must soon join the spirit world. However, he promised to return in a new form as a reminder of the peaceful brotherhood he had sought to establish among the nations.
>
> A short time after his death a new plant sprouted from his grave. This was tobacco, and it has been used in ceremonies ever since—as a symbol of unity, honesty and peace. The rising smoke from the pipe is a reminder that the thoughts and prayers of people go upward to the Creator.

American Indians view tobacco as a plant with a sacred character and use it in many ceremonies. There is no evidence that the Indians become habituated to its ceremonial use. These uses of tobacco are not recreational and many have deep religious significance.

Among the Tohono O'odham of Arizona, blowing smoke on someone is a mild form of purification. Tobacco smoke is used by the shaman to cure illness and also by those who purify someone who has been in contact with the supernatural. In the old rituals, blowing tobacco smoke was a form of prayer, which placed one in contact with the supernatural.

Among New England Indians, tobacco is a sacred plant and religious ceremonies attend the preparation of the ground and the planting of the seed.

In eastern North America, tobacco is smoked as part of prayer and of the diplomacy of receiving guests and ambassadors; used to fumigate ritually important objects such as the body of a dead chief, the body of a bear, and a sacred stone; applied to the body in solid and liquid forms as a medicine. Ascending tobacco smoke is considered an offering to the spirits, but the offering can be in solid form as well. Tobacco is tied onto a prayer stick, included in medicine bundles, burned under the hearth for the green corn ceremony, buried with the dead, deposited by waterfalls and other striking natural features, thrown into water, and deposited as an offering to the spirits of the medicinal herbs, spirits of certain game animals and crawling creatures.

Among the Delaware people, tobacco is considered a magic plant. It is offered to Kee-shay-lum-moo-kawng, and to the lesser spiritual agents called Manitowuk, as the occasion warrants. Tobacco is burned like incense in an open fire. When an herbalist gathers roots or leaves in the woods, he customarily sprinkles tobacco at the foot of the tree, or around the plant, as an offering to the spirit world. Tobacco, in addition to its many religious purposes, is used to quiet angry waters, allay destructive winds, seek good luck in hunting, return thanks to the Creator, protect a traveler, and console the bereaved.

I have seen a shaman include tobacco in his healing herbs and place it in his medicine bag. It was John Smith in the early colonial days who recognized that crossing the traditional sacred Indian tobacco with the more sturdy West Indian tobacco, produced the hybrid that resulted in the pleasant smoke which was subsequently marketed to England. The rest is history. Indian youth have as much trouble as anyone resisting the compelling ads to be cool, to smoke.

Session in Traditional Healing

Eighty people sit in a large circle. There is no front-of-the room platform, podium, projector or screen—just one very large circle with a long table at one side. On the table are an abalone shell, sage twigs, cedar boughs, a brightly colored cloth of red, yellow, black and white, a feather fan, herbs and roots. The leader is Maria Christina, from New Mexico. She tells us that her heritage is of the U.S. southwest and northern Mexico. She stands quietly by the table watching as we find seats, waiting for us to settle. She picks up a drum, taps a rhythmic and penetrating beat, calling us to a prayerful opening.

Maria Christina places sage leaves in the abalone shell and lights them. Smoke circles upward. She carries the shell in her left hand and walks around the room. In her right hand she carries the feather fan and brushes the smoke around the space—a preparatory for healing. Smoke purifies. Bad spirits are brushed away. Good spirits enter.

Maria Christina picks up each cloth and herb in turn and describes its importance to our healing. She dims the ceiling lamps and tells stories of family and heritage. Donning a tiny miner's headband light to read while the circle is engulfed in darkness, she continues. Although connected within the circle, we move into our own private caverns of thought, allowing ourselves to float into personal grief while visualizing losses. Protected by the darkness, we openly and unashamedly weep—many of us—most of us.

Allowing ample time for the tears to cleanse, Maria Christina softly tells us she will slowly raise the ceiling chandelier to full brightness. We recover our composure and return to the strength of the circle.

The next task is to select a person from the circle to share our story of grief. On the opposite side of the room, I notice a tall blonde woman. I walk across the ballroom and pull up a chair. I tell her about my pregnant teenage daughter.

"I know why you selected me" says the blonde woman. "When I was a teen, I did the same thing." Tears fill my eyes.

"It is all right for you to grieve," says the woman. "You are okay. Your daughter is okay, too." Moments later, I walk across the room and reclaim my seat.

Maria Christina asks for someone to share with the entire circle. A woman of a southwest tribe stands up and tearfully shares her story. "Thank you," says Maria Christina. "By your courage to share, you have spoken for many."

As we exit the healing session, we reach into Maria Christina's reed woven basket and retrieve a piece of root, a gift to carry away with us to continue the healing process or to share with others for their healing.

That same evening all five hundred conference goers gather for dinner, this time around individual round tables that seat ten to twelve people. There is so much talking people have to shout to the other side of the table to be heard. Dinner is followed by dancing and we dance freely until midnight, celebrating our wellness.

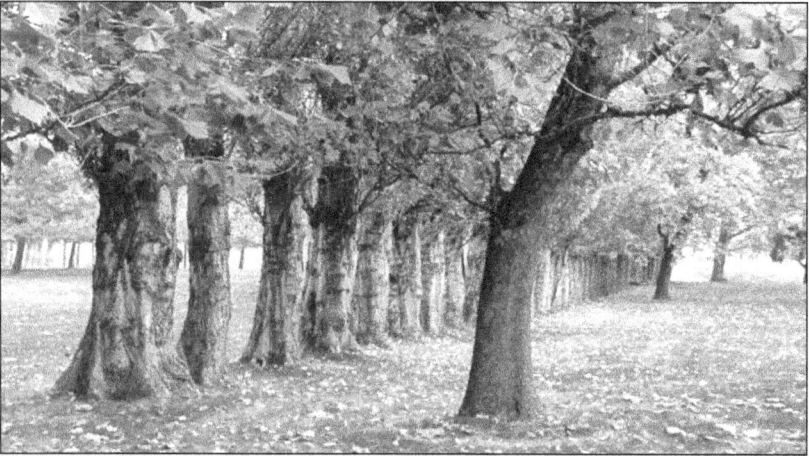

These trees face the Columbia River at Horse Thief State Park upstream from our conference in Portland. The grove is a half-mile from where *Tasgaglalah*, an ancient petroglyph and pictograph watches over the river and protects the Wishram people from disease.

April

Pangwuh?am Huhnsha? Ha

Time of the blossoms

Annual Sobriety Powwow and Dance

It is time for the annual gathering of the Cedar Bay Tribe, who have sent invitations to other tribes. Dancers from the Yakama people to the west and the Tlingit to the north come to celebrate sobriety, to dance, to listen to the wisdom of the elders, to wear ceremonial regalia, to purchase Indian crafts and pictures, to raffle handmade items and to eat Indian tacos. It is a time when elders teach the traditions to the young. It is a time that the dominant culture is invited to observe the perseverance and determination of the people to maintain sobriety, and to also see the beauty and color of the dance and to hear the haunting and rhythmic beat of the drums. I feel it is a privilege to be included.

The local high school gymnasium is the location for the annual powwow. Funding comes from tribal members, from the county self-help foundations, and from the state Division of Substance and Alcohol Abuse. Preparation for the annual sobriety powwow takes months. Artist Tom Anderson carves a wooden rattle for the raffle. Vendors bring Pendleton blankets, beaded necklaces, drums and baskets to the gathering.

All stand for the Grand Entry. Elder Native military veterans in regalia hold the United States flag and are ready to lead. Younger members carry various tribal flags. Drums beat a cadence. With dignity and sureness of foot, the procession of flags moves forward. The audience remains standing in silence as an elder veteran speaks. Children listen. Young people show respect. When the color guard retreats, the drumming intensifies and dancers take to the floor.

In regalia of feathers, shells, beads, and tin clinkers, dancers move around the room. The color, movement, and sound are mesmerizing. Long swinging tassels of the women's shawl dance hypnotize. Rhythmically swaying back and forth, the women move in a circular pattern to the beat of the drums. A few hold hands with children decked out in colorful ribbon dresses and shirts. Infants held closely by parents and grandparents join in the dance.

I slip down from the grandstand and take my two-hour shift at a long table serving Indian tacos (fry bread with beans, cheese, salad greens, and sauce), and after my stint I return to the hypnotizing drama on the dance floor.

Two tall slender handsome young men in red, blue, white, yellow and black regalia from the Tlinget nation portray the trickster Raven, using large wooden animal masks. They dance in a coat of seal fur with abalone buttons. Steathily, the dancers face each other and move around the floor. Once the legend is told, the guest Tlinget dancers leave the floor. "Fancy" dancers move in.

The regalia of one young man—a crowd favorite artisan and musician—includes eagle feathers fashioned into a bustle on his back. He dances a legend of Eagle and Raven. It is said that this particular young man prayed to the Grandfather for help in his quest to find feathers for his regalia. One day an eagle fell not far from where he was walking. He quickly, tenderly, and closely examined the fallen bird. It was dead. The young man respectfully carried the bird to the chairman for proper burial. The tribe would plan a proper interment for the eagle, and the chairman gave permission for the young man to use the feathers for regalia and dancing. The prayer and the permission to use the eagle feathers makes this young man's dance soar as if in eagle flight.

Younger dancers are bedecked in colorful ribbon shirts which parents have carefully and tenderly sewn. Powwow is a lesson in parenting, heritage and visual storytelling and connects ancestral ways of learning with the challenges of modern day diversity. The elders share their knowledge through storytelling and through dance. I realize I only need to pause and listen, caring to hear.

◆ ◆ ◆ ◆ ◆

It is spring on the campus of the University of Washington in community nursing class. One of the students demonstrates the dance that she is learning to perform for healing therapy. She brought with her two women drummers who have survived breast cancer. She invites the students of the nursing class to participate in the dance when they feel ready to do so. The drummers begin and express great joy through their drumming. The dancer begins free flowing movements which remind me of stretching exercises. She moves in a spontaneous way that speaks to how she is feeling at this moment. She passes simple drumming instruments and noisemakers to the class so we can accompany her movements. Soon others join her in dance. By the end of a few songs, most of the students and faculty are on the dance floor, moving with the rhythm of the drums. They have set aside their stress and tension and course work. They are participating in a healing dance.

◆ ◆ ◆ ◆ ◆

I have grown to love myself as a unique dancer. Dancing alone, I feel beautiful and allow the music to define the dance. I forgive my missteps of the past. Remembering the disciplined instruction of my dance teacher Lera Ray, I whisper a "thank you," as it was she who demanded perfection in the ballet and helped me to heal the noticeable limp from a broken leg. I danced the samba in the streets of Brazil. I three-stepped the two step at the Rodeo and Live Stock Show in Houston. At a health conference pow wow, I glanced at a dancer's beaded moccassined feet as she danced in her soft white deer-skin dress, placing her feet in rhythm to the drums as she moved in the circle dance. I respectfully followed and placed my feet in the same manner as she. In my own living room, with no one watching, I dance, sing, cry, and clap. I am releasing the pain and hurt, and accepting, instead, the spirit of the dance. Seeking balance, I am becoming in tune and in-step with the universe. For all of us, wherever we are and wherever we go, our journey embraces the dance.

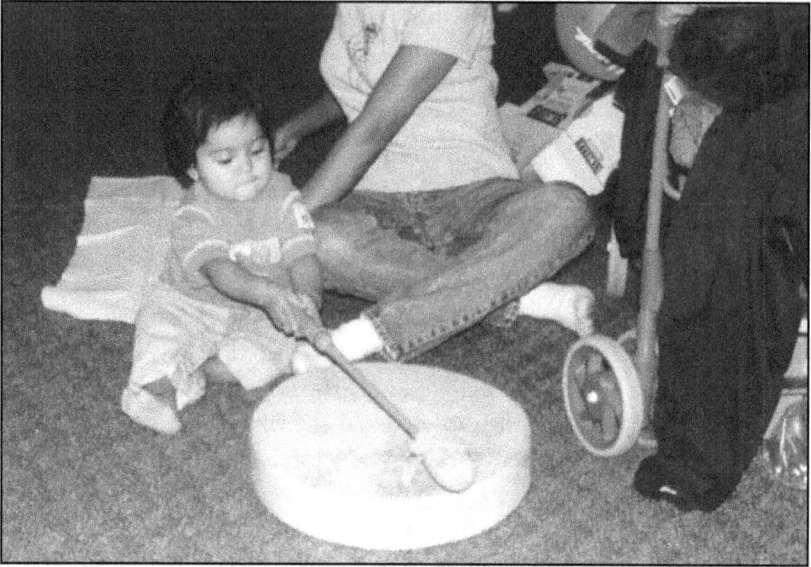

B. Young

Elders and adults teach lessons whenever there is an opportunity. I have seen infants held by parents participating in the circle dance. Rhythm, step, and beat are soothing to the infant, and places the infant in touch with the ancestors. Each culture gathers in celebration and reunion to recall and reunite with their ancestral spirits in the form of dance.

Empowerment to Say "No Alcohol"

A few health workers from outside the reservation ask if excessive alcohol use is the cause for the high rate of infant mortality. The Joint Report alludes to the possibility that alcohol could be one of the considerations. One of the women of the Focus Group says to me, "I do not drink; I do not smoke; I watch what I eat. Why did I lose my baby?" But a few of the women in the Focus Group are in recovery. Outside of this small circle, I have little information.

At the annual meeting of the American Public Health Association, an eastern Cherokee receives the association's prestigious Excellence Award. Before a crowd of five thousand people, this impressive woman, the first Native American nurse to receive a Ph.D. from the University of California, speaks of the adverse effects of alcohol on the future of the Native American family. She said that there is not an Indian reservation or tribe in the country that does not have an alcohol awareness program trying to change individual behavior as well as public perceptions.

While working for the Washington State Department of Health setting up prenatal care access programs, I read *The Broken Cord* by Michael Dorris, which helped me to understand Fetal Alcohol Syndrome/Fetal Alcohol Effects (FAS/FAE). The book provides an opportunity to understand the power and devastation of an invasive chemical, known as a teratogen, or "monster-causing toxin." The chemical, poison to the system, is alcohol. Dorris adopted a child from the Pine Ridge Sioux Reservation without knowing the prenatal history of the birth mother, who had died of alcohol poisoning. At the time of the adoption, information on FAS/FAE was not well known. His story helped medical professionals understand the devastation of this disease and moved many to be advocates for not drinking during pregnancy. Not only must the mother-to-be observe what she eats and drinks, but the father, too, is alerted to be aware that what he eats and drinks is important in the formation of a new fetus.

As a white nurse in Indian country, and an invited guest on the reservation, it is not for me to initiate a discussion of alcohol intake or use. Stereotypes about Indians and alcohol are offensive and damaging.

The community health representative and a tribal elder instruct me to sit and watch a video of the Alkali Lake tribe in Canada. Both women went to the Alkali Lake training to promote healthy behavior around drinking. In the video, tribal members act out their own stories of abuse, violence, fights and confrontations with the booze promoter who pushed drinking behavior. Tribal members learn empowerment and say "no!" to any more drinking on tribal lands. This is the story of a tribe with an alcoholism rate close to 100%, and their children were beginning to copy the behaviors of the drinking adults. One tribal member said, "This must end. We are destroying ourselves and our future," and she changed her behavior. She convinced her husband to do the same and together they convinced others. Slowly, the drinking behavior changed. The tribe reversed its former alcoholism rate and is now almost 100% sober. What would happen in the dominant white community if we said "no" as well and led our children on a no-alcohol path?

May

Panjulashxuhtltu

Time when blueback return

Storyteller

She comes to the tribal center rather like St. Nicholas—with a pack on her back. In the middle of the second floor office lobby, the storyteller dumps the contents of the pack and then stands back to admire one hundred stuffed bunnies of various shapes and colors and degrees of wear, lying in a heap on the floor. Gingerly, the storyteller approaches the huge pile, bends and tenderly picks up each and describes its character to the mental health social worker, and me.

"You two," the storyteller directs, "pick out forty bunnies for our discussion downstairs and help me pack 'em down. After all, isn't this evening's entertainment what you might call *Evening out at the Oyster Shell?*"

We do as directed. The community gathering takes place in the Georgetown Room under the eyes of the portrait gallery of Native ancestors and under the large cedar board painting, *Trail of the Spirits*, depicting the even more watchful eyes of Spirit Moon. The storyteller, a master of the art from the Aleutian Islands, begins her tales as soon as the tribal members and their invited non-native neighbors from near-by towns are settled to hear.

To the delight of children and adults alike, the large bunny bag is dumped on the floor in the middle of the room. One by one, the storyteller picks out a bunny, describes its character, and places it in a circle on the floor. "This one looks a bit tipsy. He stopped by the saloon on his way home from work." Another bunny is selected from the pile. "This bunny likes to drink. That's why her eyes are so sad." That bunny becomes part of the circle. She reaches for another bunny. And then another. All become part of the enlarging circle. The storyteller turns to the gathered group. "Do you see this circle? It is the community I grew up in. I know these characters. They are my family, friends and neighbors." Among the listeners there are knowing nods.

The storyteller pauses, bends down, and—with bunnies flying into the air—breaks up the bunny circle community. Bunnies are again in a confused heap on the floor. Their former circle community has been disorganized. The bunnies are now free to take on new identities. The storyteller looks at the gathered guests. "It is your turn to tell a story. Come. Select a bunny and tell the bunny's story." Eagerly, the listeners come forward to claim a bunny. Chairs are moved into smaller circles of five or six, and the meeting room begins to hum with several stories being told at once. Within the smaller story circles, the bunnies become daring divers of the deep, a tiny bunny lost in a woodpile, a grandparent bunny that is going to boarding school and a tiny brother bunny.

All too quickly, the evening is ending. Bunnies return to the center of the room. The adoptive parent smudges the bunny by holding it close and passing it over the light of a candle set beside the packing bag. A silent prayer is offered as the bunny is safely and tenderly tucked back into the carrying bag for the trip home.

Feeling quite smug that I was responsible for the successful *Evening Out at the Oyster Shell*, I arrive at the health clinic staff meeting the next morning ready to hear just how wonderful, creative and insightful I was to engage the native storyteller. After the routine agenda of the health clinic, we open the comment section. Out comes anger. I am soundly criticized for the previous evening's program. I sit stunned, unable to respond. What did I overlook? What am I doing here anyway? Why is it taking me so long to understand?

The health clinic staff meeting adjourns. I hustle to my office on the second floor, shut the door, and sit in misery. Was it arrogance to think that I should bring a storyteller to the tribe? Had I been too possessive because my program grant facilitated the evening discussion? Why was I criticized so severely? Reaching for the phone, I dial the storyteller. She answers on the second ring.

"*Evening Out at the Oyster Shell* brought the tribe an evening of outside entertainment. It also brought the opportunity for introspection and reflection," she explained. "When I described the characters in my own community, they saw their family members and themselves in those characters. It is a painful process to begin to see yourself as you are; it is painful to see the truth."

"But why me?" I ask. "Why do I have to take the heat for this? I feel terrible."

She continued, "Because you brought a program that gives us all the opportunity to see ourselves, and we do not want to see the dark part of ourselves. We would rather that remain hidden. You are the outsider. It is easy to place the blame on you. Maybe you'll just go away and not cause any more pain."

Reflecting on all this, I consider the presence of alcohol in my own life. I grew up not knowing alcohol except for the bottle of whiskey on the top shelf that was fetched for Granddad's "hot toddy" when he had a sore throat. The recipe was one capful of whiskey to one cup of boiling water to one teaspoon of honey. Granddad's toddy cured anything, or at least you forgot about the sore throat.

When my daughters were five and two, my marriage broke up due to my husband's drinking and unpredictable behavior. Two years later, I married a man who I thought was a step up. He was. Up from the cheap large bottles of wine brought by students for intellectual discussion to much finer brands. The addiction to cigarettes from husband number one moved to fine Cuban cigars in husband number two. Number two's other addictions included gambling and sex. I did not trade up in marriage partners. I traded into more intensely addictive behaviors.

The storyteller caused the oyster shell to pry open. The pile of bunnies in a huge heap in the middle of the floor carried not only the participants' stories; but mine as well. I begin to understand the anger.

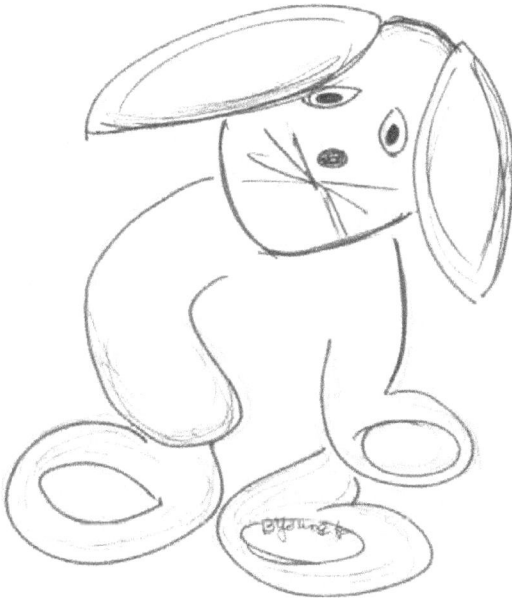

Pharmacology Class

I help the medicine woman carry her plants to the classroom. As we walk, she sees the red clover trampled underfoot. "That clover," she says, "would be useful for sore throats and colds. It is so easy to get; it is here at our feet."

Sitting in a relaxed, calm circle of Native American women, we are eager to hear the pharmacology lecture from the medicine woman. She learned her skills not from a textbook, but from tribal knowledge passed down through the generations. In many tribes, the medicine person is carefully selected and trained for this position. Medicine women learn and understand the potent properties of plants used in healing.

She stands behind a table that holds her plants. She picks up the first plant. "This is yarrow. It is used for arthritis. You use the whole plant. For headaches, you would chew the tops. For diarrhea, you use the roots. It is an instant cure. For hair rinse, use the whole plant."

She picks up another plant. "This is the madrona plant. It is used for diarrhea." Next is devil's club, "good for sinus." A woman in the circle says her tribe uses this plant for dandruff. The medicine woman says that devil's club can be boiled and inhaled for rheumatism. Also used for rheumatism are: elder bark, alder bark, cherry, cascain, and chitum.

To prepare skunk cabbage, "Place the leaf in boiling water and then apply as a poultice directly on an area experiencing pain."

"Hawthorne berry is good for the heart."

"From yew tree bark you get a cure for cancer. You might mix it with Canadian moss."

"Native huckleberry is used as a blood purifier and in the treatment of diabetics. For high blood pressure you mix with oak bark. In preparation, you boil the whole stalk."

"Eucalyptus is used in colds, flu, and congestion."

"Honeysuckle..." I write as fast as I can, trying not to miss an important detail of the preparation or the cure or the intent for giving. She doesn't wait for me to catch up but keeps on explaining.

"Peppermint is used for upset stomach. It also helps to relax you when you are tired."

"Chamomile is a relaxant." I flash back to Beatrix Potter's story of Peter Rabbit who ate too many carrots and vegetables in Mr. McGregor's garden and narrowly escaped with his life. When Peter hurriedly ran home, his delight in filching all of those tender vegetable plants was gone. He was sick and his mother put him to bed with chamomile tea.

"Red clover is used for colds."

"Dandelion is an energy tea. It is a blood purifier and cleans the kidneys. Use the roots."

"Plantain is a medicine for cancerous sores. It is excellent for healing. You make a drink."

"Licorice fern is a tea for sore throat. You use the root. I have known it to be effective for cancer of the throat."

"Wild strawberry is a good healing plant. The runners can be used in making a heart medicine. The leaves are good for pregnancy. They help in a successful delivery."

The class is attentive and connected. Some share their own tribal wisdom and pharmacology practices. An elder from a tribe on the coast speaks. "The spoon leaf and squirrel tail draw out infection. I remember when my son's arm and toe became infected and swollen. The leaves of these plants were chopped and crushed and braised in warm water and then applied directly to the infection which was then wrapped with an ace bandage. In two days, the swelling was down and the infection was gone. He was healed." This same elder goes on to say. "I think that the county trucks spray the road side to keep the plants back, and now I can't find these plants."

Another woman speaks. "*Uk muk* is horsetail and makes a tea that is good for diabetics."

"Our tribe uses crabapple tea for arthritis," says a woman who is speaking for the first time.

The medicine woman saves the best for last: a columbine plant. "This is important in love, and I am not giving you the formula." She has a twinkle in her eye, passes the plant to me and says, "I want a report in six months." Class is dismissed.

Carefully, I transport my columbine plant home and place it in the garden by my back door. I count off the months—July, August, September, October, November and December. I must report to the medicine woman in December.

◆ ◆ ◆ ◆ ◆

I remember my pharmacology class and a heavy blue textbook, circa 1962. It was quite a feat to master all the information contained between the covers of that book. As nursing students, we lived in fear from our demanding instructor who met us on the medical floor well before 6:00 a.m. each day. We were to respond to each drug question she asked. "What medication is your patient receiving? Why? How will the medicine affect the body? On what organism will it be effective? How is the medicine administered? How will it be taken? Is it a pill or capsule? An injection? A suppository? Is it to be given intravenously? What are the side effects? What are the complications? What is the duration of the effect? For how long is the medicine to be taken—days, weeks, months?" We students knew it cold. If I were to look through that old blue pharmacology book of the 60s today, would I find similarities to the lecture of the medicine woman? Would the information in the blue text reflect any of her ancient knowledge?

The columbine is important for love.

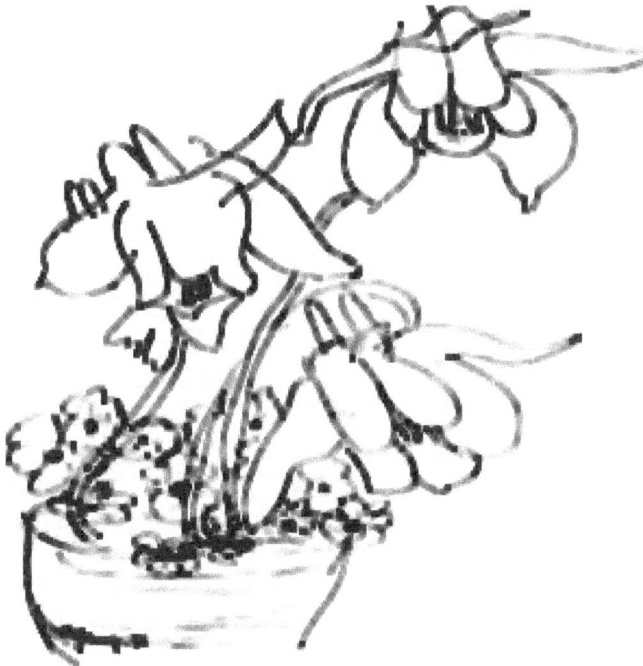

Sweat Lodge

Deep among the trees in walking distance from the Long House, a sweat lodge is being built. Long curved poles are latticed together into a domed structure over a sizable pit in which hot rocks will be placed. Tarps and wool blankets are placed over the dome to keep heat and steam within. Sprinkling water over the hot rocks in the center pit makes steam. The structure resembles a womb. The sweat lodge is a ritual of cleansing, of purification, of sweating out the old and the pain. It is a sacred practice.

A fire of rocks and logs is built just outside the entrance to the sweat lodge. The leader places the rocks and logs in preparation for the sweat. When all is ready, she offers prayers and directs us to enter the lodge. As a non-native, I ask if it is appropriate for me to enter the sweat lodge; there is "stuff" that I need to sweat out of my system. The leader leaves the decision to me. I decide to sweat.

The women entering the sweat lodge gather around the outside fire. We lift the Pendleton blanket door flap and enter, crawling on our hands and knees around the stone pit to sit in a circle surrounding it. Cedar boughs cover the floor of the lodge. My friend from another tribe bends down upon entering the lodge, as is her tribal custom, and offers a kiss to Mother Earth. It reminds me of the heads of state who—when returning to their native country—bend down and kiss the earth. We sit in the dark as the leader drums, prays and asks for the hot rocks to be deposited in the inside pit. Glowing hot rocks are carried through the flap and placed in the pit. In the darkness of our shared space, the rocks glow with warmth. When water is sprinkled on the rocks, steam hisses and circles upward. We breathe deeply and allow our bodies to feel the heat. We relax and accept the healing powers of this place. More rocks are added to the pit. More water is sprinkled; steam rises and fills the lodge.

After a time, the leader begins to hum a melodic song. We join her and soon the sweat lodge is a harmonious chorus. Eventually, we end our meditations and crawl out into a lovely dark night, illuminated only by the glowing embers of the log fire. We feel cleansed, purified, lighter, loved and whole. Through this sweating process, we emerge from the womb reborn.

We quietly and reverently douse the last sparks of the wood fire, pick up our towels and carefully—with the few flashlights among us—walk through the forest to our cabins and bunks. A million diamonds in the sky brighten our path. It is close to midnight. Back at the cabin, I quietly climb into my down sleeping bag on the lower bunk so as not to disturb the sleeping women.

◆ ◆ ◆ ◆ ◆

In the morning as I let the warm waters of my city shower flow over me, I am reminded of the long showers we took in our hotel rooms in Bahia, Brazil, in 1967. I had been assigned to public health work on the edge of the *sertao*, a dusty, brush and low tree region in the interior of the state of Bahia. For the annual conference, the Peace Corps volunteers gathered in the state capital of Salvador. Living for a few days in a hotel room was luxury. Having a real shower with hot and cold water was a true gift. In our assigned town of Ibicarai, I heated a pan of water on my propane stove and took a sponge bath. My husband was able to stand scantily clothed under the roof gutter and allow the rainwater to pour over him.

There, in Salvador, Bahia, hotel shower waters washed away the dust and the dirt and the past year's troubles. I felt reborn then, as well. I remember.

June

Pankwuhla

Time of the salmonberries

Canoe

The Cedar Bay people are descendants of the Canoe People. Skilled in the ways of the ocean, they canoed the tributaries of the Columbia, navigating between ocean and bay. Large canoes were built for many members of the tribe with small simple dugouts for solo fishing in the streams. Historically, when a tribal member died, she was placed in her own canoe along with her tools. The canoe was then placed high in the trees or on posts to offer good passage as the deceased paddled into the next life.

The Canoe People enjoyed a bounty of food—fish from the rivers, shellfish from the shores; salmon and bottom fish such as sturgeon were limitless. Even in their diminished numbers, fish continue to give. When a Cedar Bay tribal member takes the life of a great fish or the first fish of a new season, he gives thanks and blesses the spirit of the fish that feeds his family. Historically, canoes were used not only to obtain food but in celebration of great events such as weddings and namings. They were used to visit other tribes in celebration or for trade.

The Chinook nation developed a great reputation for trading, going far up the coast to Alaska and south along the coast to Northern California. Chinooks traded inland as well with the nearby Chehalis and east across the mountains with the Yakama. A Chinook trade language was developed.

Lewis and Clark came on the Jefferson expedition at the same time and in the same region where the Hudson Bay Company was establishing outposts for trade. Both the expedition and the trading posts opened the area for exploration and settlement by non-natives. White trappers and settlers soon followed in great numbers. Communicable diseases came along with them. Tribes along the rivers and streams became sick. A few Indian survivors retreated to their canoes and paddled to the coast. Great and healthy nations of families living among the abundance of the forests and waters were decimated by diseases for which they had no immunity.

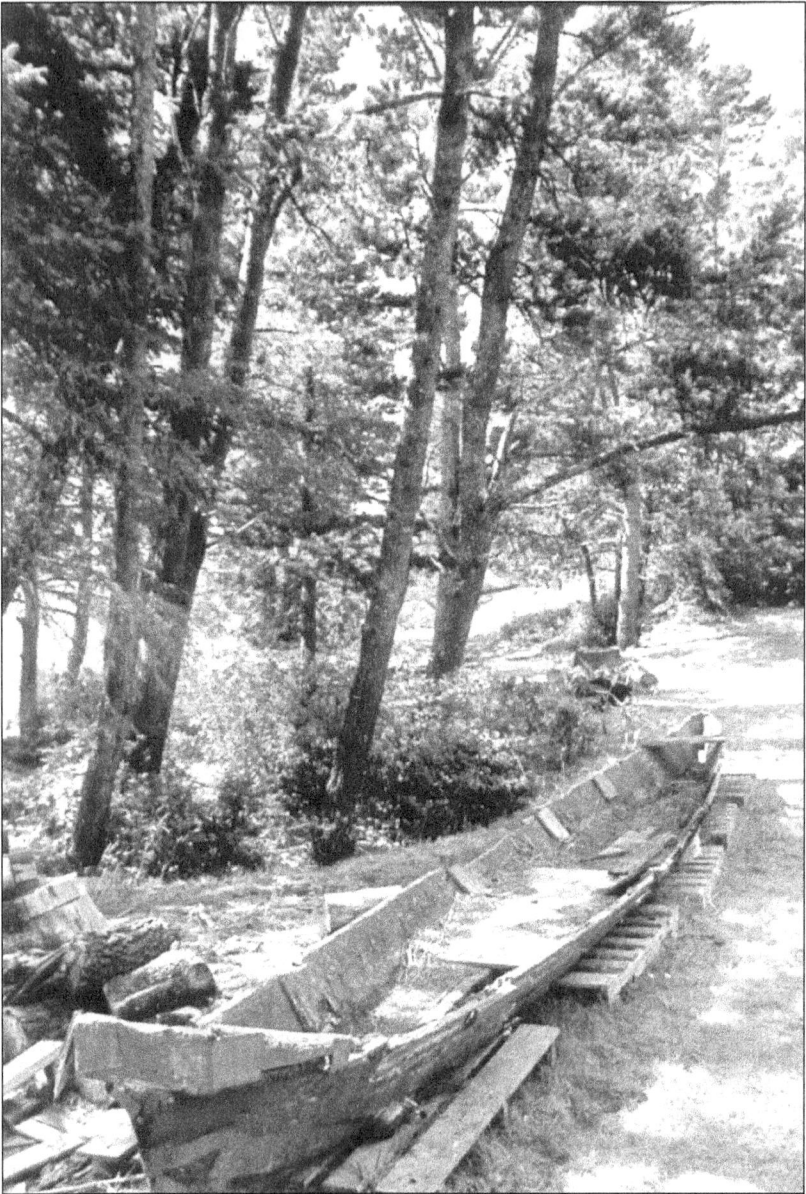

A few survivors retreated to the tide flats, the shoalwaters. Their canoes, once the pride of the waterways, disappeared as many of their ancestors had. Sturgeon, salmon and shellfish diminished as well.

◆ ◆ ◆ ◆ ◆

In the weeks after my arrival at the reservation, I hear rumors that a small independent logging company is planning to give the tribe a very large western red cedar log to be made into a canoe to be used by present-day tribal members. There is much anticipation. In the past the ancestors formed a circle around the chosen tree. Prayers were given and the tribe asked permission that the spirit of the tree be transferred to the spirit of the canoe. The spirit of the tree would continue to serve and guard the people by becoming a strong seaworthy canoe through the effort and skill of the tribe. This was the old way.

Times are different. The lands are no longer communally used and respected. They are divided into plots and privately owned. Large, corporate and sometimes absentee logging companies—some as far away as England—own the lands.

A young Cedar Bay tribal artist carves a model of the canoe he plans to make from the giant log. He will use the ancient methods—carving primarily with an adze. The cedar tree will be felled by company loggers and trucked to the reservation. The tribe will have to forgo the traditional tree blessing in the forest, but they will conduct an appropriate ceremony when the log arrives. The tree will receive its blessing.

The day finally comes when the massive cedar log is hauled to the reservation and placed in the field where the canoe carver will work. On the day of the celebration, the tribal spiritual leader leads the blessing. Meanwhile, my daughter hooks her bicycle to the metal frame of a bus three counties away and then pedals the last ten miles to the reservation. As she rounds the bend in sight of the field, tribal members and guests are circling the cedar.

The shaman beats a welcome rhythm on the drum, which calls us to gather in the presence of the great log. As we stand in quiet respect, the shaman sings to the Great Spirit of praise for the day, for the life of this tree from the forest, for the people who will touch this log and carve the canoe and for all of those who will ride in it in the future. He cleanses the log by smudging. When the prayers are complete, he asks us to place our hands on the log to give it energy. He instructs people to feel the energy of the log in return and to take its energy as it is offered.

As I lay my hands upon the log, I pray this will be a tribal journey of renewed health and an awakening of the heritage and culture that brought these people to this place. I relinquish my strict Eurocentric thinking and place myself with the spirit of the shaman and the cedar log.

Following the blessing ceremony, tribal members and guests walk to the community center and Long House for celebration. A dinner of salmon, Dungeness crab, chowder, corn, salad and Rose's famous berry cobbler are gratefully consumed. This celebration of the log symbolizes the return of the Canoe people.

◆ ◆ ◆ ◆ ◆

I am remembering my first canoe experience. It was at the National Cash Register Old River Recreation Park in Dayton, Ohio, in the 50s where my mother took me to learn to swim, canoe and enjoy Sunday evening band concerts played by area high school students. I remember the "J" stroke of stern paddling, pulling toward you along the side of the canoe and then swinging out away. I learned how to tandem paddle, solo paddle, how to right the canoe and how to turn and get out of dense growth. I later taught these canoeing skills to young girl scouts at Camp Whippoorwill, located a short distance from Fort Ancient—home to burial mounds of the Hopewell and Adena Peoples. It was there that I remember searching creek beds for trilobite and fern fossils, remnants of a pre-glacial geography of ancient lakes. It was on the girl scout canoeing trips that we would sing this song to the rhythm of paddle strokes....

> Dip, dip and swing.
> Dip, dip and swing her back
> Flashing with silver
> Smooth as the wild goose flight,
> Dip, dip and swing.
> Dip, dip and swing.

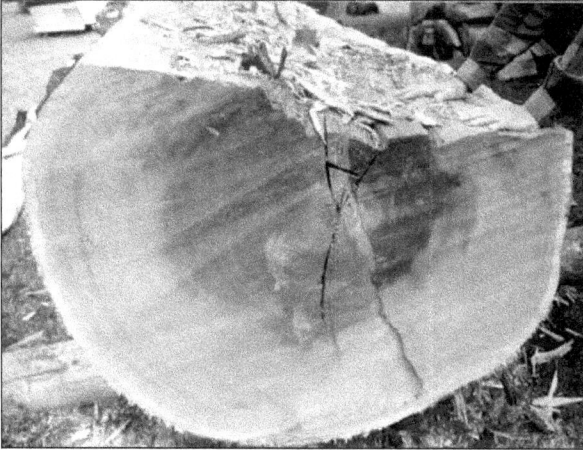

Cecelia Kayano

Laboring Upstream

Like the salmon, I seem to be swimming upstream against the current. I am having a tough time leaping over the rocks. Here I am—a nurse with a master's degree in health planning. I have experience with state programs. I have credentials. I have communication skills. Why am I laboring? I know that I have a good program and that I am the appropriate choice to lead this program. Why do the grant administrators not understand my communications? Why am I being made to jump through hoops? Why is the health program, which I thought "culturally sensitive" to a fault, not accepted by funders in the other Washington?

To my angst, the chairman responds simply, "Now, Barbara, you know what it is to be Indian."

That hurts. The success of my program has nothing to do with education or talent. It has everything to do with image, prejudice, fear, control… and politics.

The chairman says, "You are currently going in circles with only one paddle. You must feel the current and the presence of the paddle in the water. You must sight your course and flow forward."

My co-worker, the one who led the women to the clinic for breast exams, places in my hand a gift. It is a small wooden hand-carved paddle with a green bead attached. It is a connection, between the Canoe people of the coast and a nurse from the city.

Holding my tiny paddle, I decide to stop going in circles, to correct the course of the health promotion program and to paddle hard upstream.

I seek the ancient wisdom of the Canoe people.

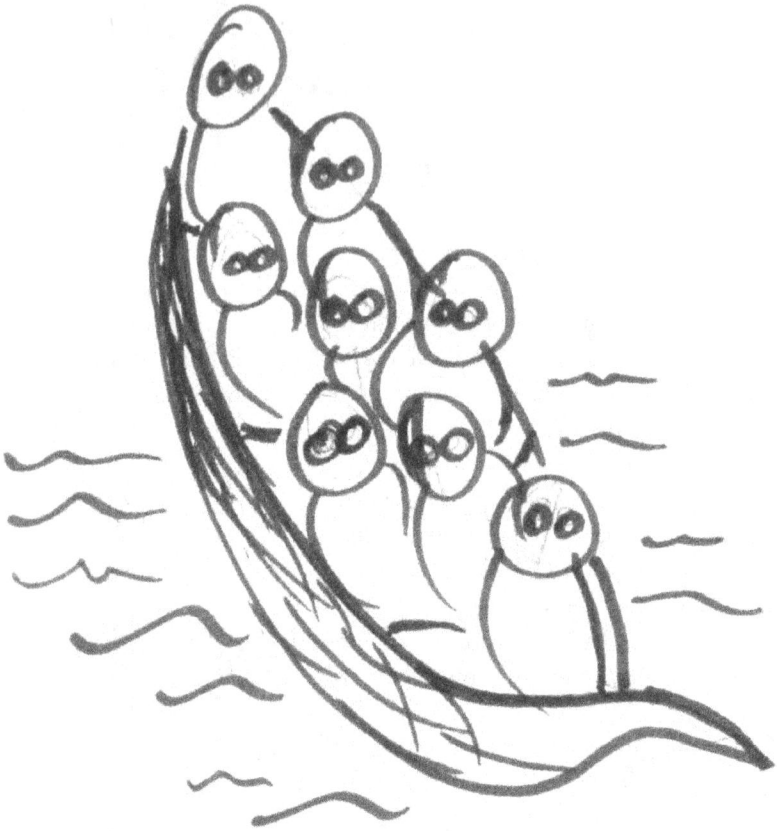

"Shimmering Down From the Sky" was a 1997 mask and sculpture exhibit at the downtown Vancouver Art Museum in British Columbia. A large sculpture in the middle of the hall depicted a hunting canoe with eight masked and robed figures, who represented ancestors of the Canoe People.

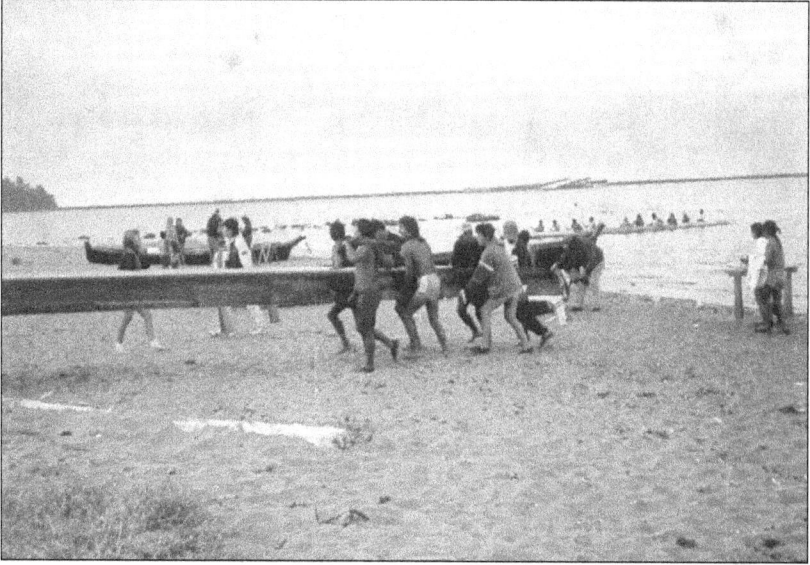

In the most northwest point of the country, along the coast from the Canoe People of Cedar Bay are the descendants of the Great Whalers. The Makah celebrate their heritage with annual canoe races. Drummers on shore beat the rhythm for their canoe team. Salmon filets set upright on latticed sticks are cooked over alder logs on the beach. Children play nearby using logs as teeter-totters or as jump-off places.

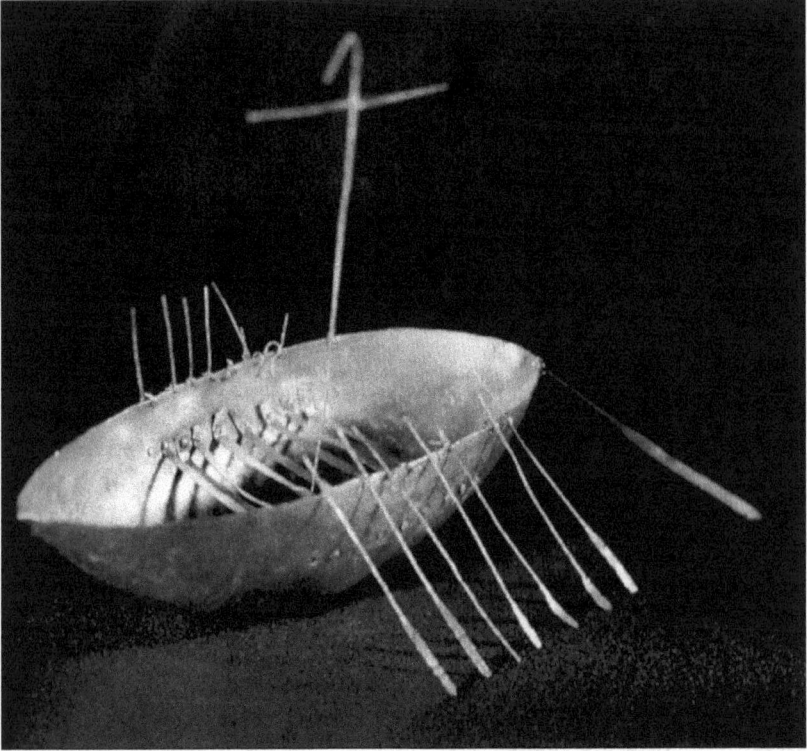

This ancient Irish boat model made in gold is a miniature—complete with benches, mast and oars. It may have been an offering to a water deity such as the Irish Sea God, Manannan. Broighter, County Derry, Ireland; dated to the first century BCE.

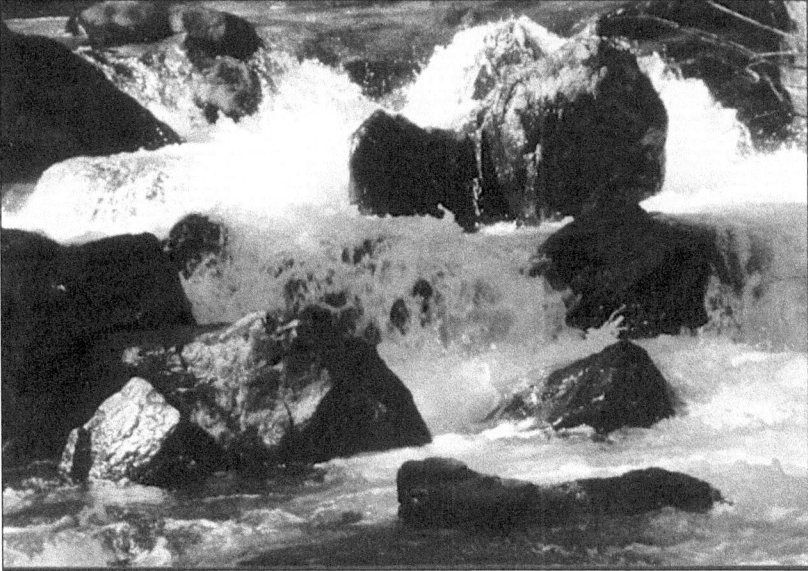

Facing an upstream swim against the rapids and jumping the boulders seems overwhelming, yet the salmon do it. They are swimming to reach their birthplace to deposit eggs and sperm for the next generation. They are given the will, spirit and energy to succeed. Their decaying carcasses replenish the earth.

The Givaway

The community health representative, who was on many occasions responsible for my orientation to the tribal community, walked past my office door muttering, "It's been a year since Kenny's death. It's time for a Giveaway."

"What is a Giveaway?" I ask.

"It is a time of remembrance, a memorial to commemorate the life of the one who has died. After a year of mourning has passed, you gather together the family and friends and give away the possessions of the one who has died. You share the spirit of the loved one with those who have gathered. All carry the person's spirit away with them."

A few months later the tribal community, family and friends of four other deceased tribal members gather for a memorial. The dead include the mother and father of the tribal chairman, a young man who was a veteran, and the son of one of the members of the basket circle.

I feel honored to be asked to participate and sit in the last row. Relatives and friends come from all over the area. Although it has been more than one year since these deaths, the gathering gives the family members permission to speak of their relatives. Pictures are shared. Stories are told. Possessions of the deceased are brought forward and given away. Handmade gifts are distributed to guests. My friend from the basket circle walks back to me and hands me a necklace that she made—white bone, black and deep green glass beads separated by tiny gold beads. She said I will help to carry the spirit of her son.

◆ ◆ ◆ ◆ ◆

I call the graduating nursing students together into a circle and ask them to contribute to a giveaway table. Placing my daughter's handmade post cards on the table, I softly begin to cry. My daughter left that morning for school in Scotland, and I am already missing her. Students come forward to place items on the table. One puts a card with a quote from her grandmother that she reads every morning. It helps her get through the tough days at school. Another lays her dictionary on the table to help a fellow student in the same course. The next student brings a picture of a puffin because it represents many pleasurable hours with her son. Another places colored markers. Another, a leather pouch that contained a piece of crystal. Another, three chocolate bars for quick energy. Each, in turn, makes a contribution to the table. Then, the gifts are distributed, each to whom it is supposed to go. The students leave the room, the class and the university with a shared spirit.

July

Panklaswhas

Time to gather native blackberries

Cultural Transition

The commute from home to work on the reservation is approximately two hours—crossing rivers, driving through the forest, concentrating on the road instead of the waves of the Pacific Ocean and the rocky side of Willapa Bay to the tide waters. I need the time to think, meditate and plan. Whether I am going from home to the reservation or from the reservation home, I always need the full two hours to put my work and life into perspective.

A subpoena was hand delivered to my home. The hearing for child support for my daughter would be heard in Houston, Texas on July 12. I am expected to be present. Yet, this is the same date I am to give the next draft of my work plan to the grant administrator in Washington, D.C. I cannot afford the trip to Houston, but I need the court to rule in my favor. My professional colleagues at the tribal center advise an alternative. "Do something special for yourself," they said. "You do not need to travel to Houston. Allow the process to take care of it."

Near closing time at the tribal center, the evening of July 11, two native teachers from Bay Center stop to visit. They speak of the sacred grove of old growth cedar trees on Long Island in the bay. Many of their tribal ancestors fled to the island to escape the communicable diseases that were decimating Columbia River tribes. Intently, I listen. I, too, want a retreat to survive my emotional and financial crises. When the teachers leave the center, I call the only person I know who can take me to the island—a former tug boat captain who tours visitors in the waters around Nahcatta and Willapa Bay. It is already well past five o'clock.

"Do you have any bookings for tomorrow morning?" I ask the captain.

"No, I'm available."

"Will you take me to Long Island?" I plead.

"It depends entirely upon the tides," he responds. He goes on to explain the nautical terms, another language to me.

Calculating quickly, I ask myself, do I have the right to go? Would

143

I be violating sacred Indian ground? Who should I tell that I am going?

"I'll meet you at the dock." I blurt before I lose my nerve. Tomorrow is Friday. To seem irresponsible is not in my heritage. To be efficient and worthy of time is. I inform my two colleagues that, indeed, I am taking their advice and doing something for myself. Completely forgetting about the work plan deadline, I put in for personal leave. Since the administrative staff has already left the building, I do not receive permission. Instead of standing in a court of law in hot Houston, I will be boating to an isolated island to seek the wisdom of the ancient cedars. I close my office door behind me, walk quickly to the parking lot and drive out to the highway that takes me south along the bay. It takes two hours of curvy driving around inlets and sloughs to reach the peninsula point where we will embark in the morning, according to the tides.

Early the next morning the captain and I prepare lunches, jackets and gear. The phone rings: my daughter. "Your boss wants you to call. You have a report due in Washington." I had completely forgotten.

"Thanks, honey. I'll take care of it. It was good of you to call." I hang up the phone and quickly dial the tribal chairman. I level with my boss about what I am doing.

"They want the next draft of the work plan. I wish that you would have told me earlier what you were doing. I would have been better prepared when they called."

"I'm sorry," I respond.

"Ask for an extension. That will cover you."

"Thank you for understanding." I hang up the phone.

I need to fax a request for extension to Washington so that they will have it today. I am two hours from the office at a small dock in a tiny oyster village on the bay side of a peninsula that juts out into the Pacific Ocean. I have no typewriter, but the captain has a fax machine. I hand write the extension request and send the fax. Then, I call to be certain that it arrived and is dated July 12th. We grab the last of our gear and head to the dock.

The boat slowly disengages from the mooring and we sputter over to the gasoline dock before heading out into bay waters. Facing the wind directly, I grip the rail to steady myself. The wind blows my hair back and I allow tension to go with the wind. The captain is in control. I let it all go and relax with the movement.

When we reach the island, the captain slowly motors in and drops anchor. I am instructed to "prepare to beach." I take off my shoes and socks, roll up my jeans, and slide out into the water. My feet touch smooth pebbles, the size of quarters. I grab the back pack and wade to shore. The captain secures the boat and grips a long line that he shoulders to shore. He tethers the boat to a tree. I re-sock and shoe, unroll jeans, sling on the backpack and follow the captain to the grove. We speak softy of boats and water, but fall silent as we near the grove.

Upon entering the ancient grove, I whisper a prayer of thanks. I am in a sacred place, a place of quiet, of reverence, of history—of wisdom. I feel it engulf and comfort me. I sense the freedom to be who I am. I sense a history not without pain, but of survival and permanence. I look up to see the tops of these great trees. I look up and up and up. I lean against a tree and feel the rough ridges in its bark. When I look up as high as I can see, there are brilliant rays of sunlight coming through the top branches. I decide to circumnavigate just one tree, walking around and around. Then, I walk the path through the forest, enjoying each tree I meet. I climb over fallen and rotting branches that nourish the forest environment.

I come to tree stumps cut many years ago. Loggers' footholds are higher up than I can reach on tiptoe. These are magnificent trunks—providing still a sense of strength and permanence. It must have been the early practice to cut selectively, because now I can still enjoy old growth cedars that offer a place of needed refuge.

I select a magnificent cedar, a chief tree among others, a dignified grandfather. I am quiet. I listen. I am present. I have brought my troubles here. I remain quiet and continue to listen to the forest and to the wisdom of the old growth. After a time, I pick up my backpack and continue my walk through the grove. I am at peace, leaving my stress, my worry and my concern in the forest. Child support will be resolved.

I am quieter on the way back to the boat and feel lighter. Before I remove my socks and shoes on the beach, I bend to pick up several stones. Rolling up my jeans and wading to the boat, I climb over the side and prepare for disengaging from the shore. As we pull the anchor aboard, I am aware of the change in the water level. Our timing is just right. Any longer on the island and we would have had to stay the night. We cautiously turn the boat and head back. When the motor reaches cruising hum, I unwrap the lunches. We feast.

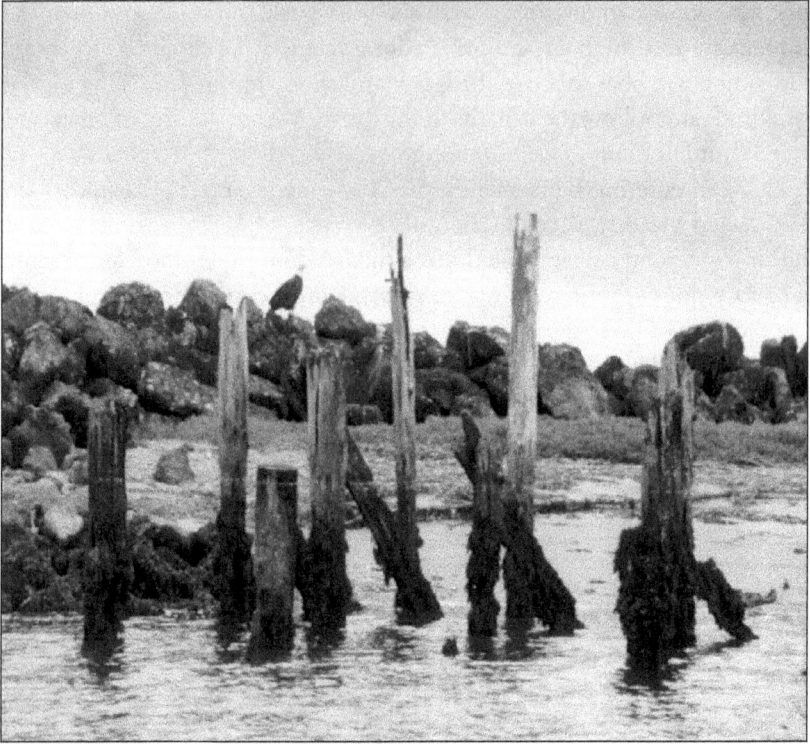

A bald eagle, standing sentry to the port, observes our departure for the island.

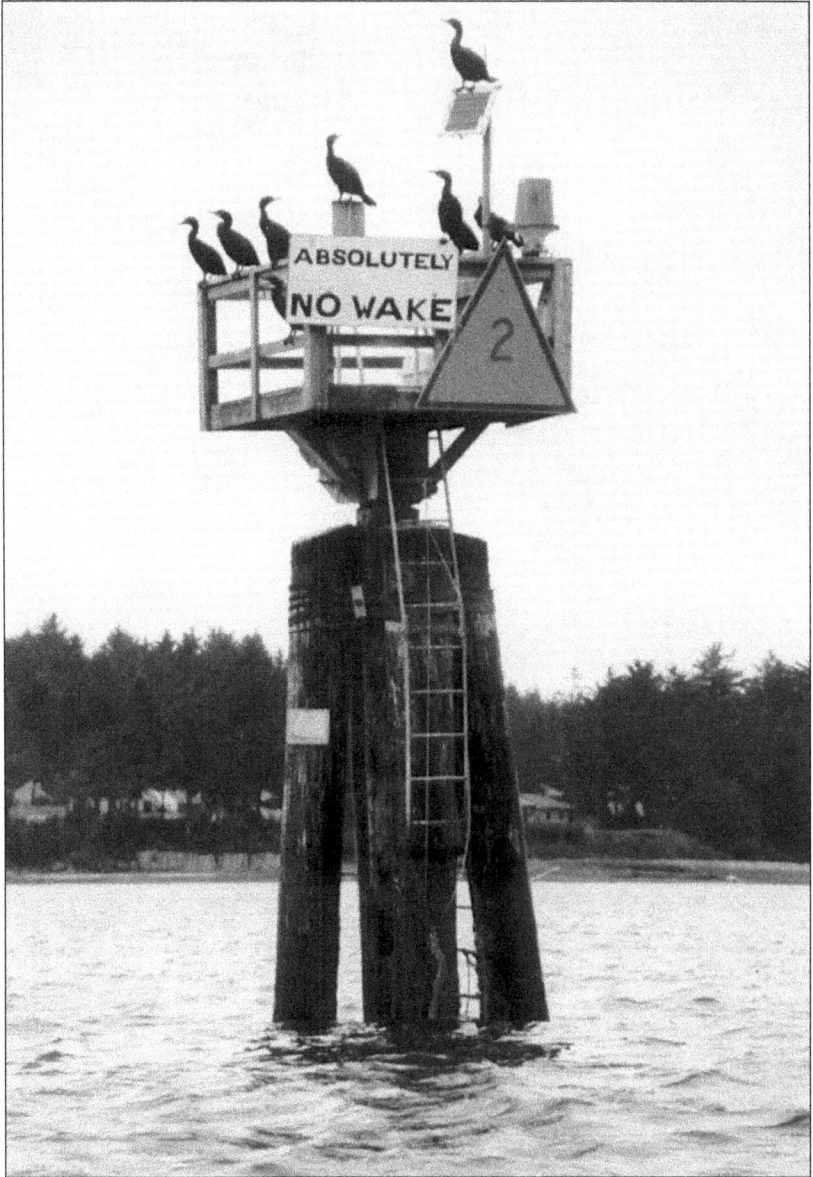

Circles, Tree and Me

Life is a circle from birth to old age to childhood again;
Sun rises and moves in a circular direction during the course of the day;
Glass from which I drink is circular;
Seeds to plant for spring sprout upward;
Tree is round, strong, and reaches to the sun;
I put our arms around Tree, encircle it with love.

Tree is center of circle
Grows upward and downward;
Receives nourishment from
East
South
West
North
Begins as seed
Grows to old age
Returns
Replenishes the earth.

I am center of circle
Look outward
Up
Down
East
South
West
North
Seven Sacred Directions

Circle is healing journey. As I move, circle expands
Meet new people; new horizons are envisioned
Feel unity with sisters of another nation
Kinship with forests through which I pass
Trees sharing quiet wisdom.

When I see stacked logging trucks, I wish trees well on their final journey.
When I see fresh jagged trunks, torn with unsharpened scissors, I feel their injuries.
We share sun and moon, warmth and cold.
We live together.

Circles of respect, honesty, hope and health are messages of my story.
Relationship with each other and with the land.
No sharp corners

Energy flows from inside out
From outside in.
We are connected to all others—human, animal, environment—the earth.
All related.

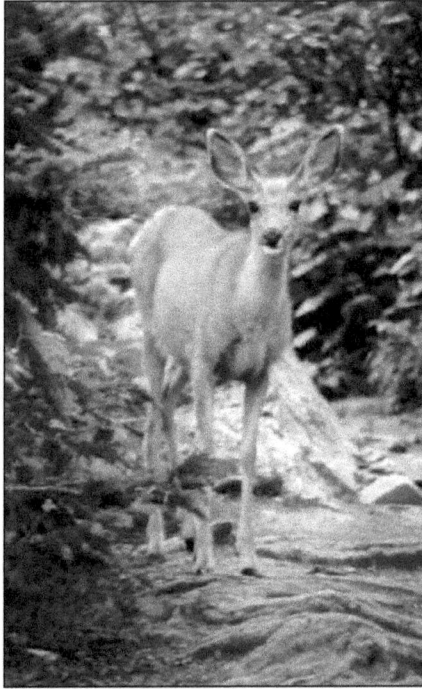

A deer moved out of her protective forest cover to meet me on the path.
She reminded me of what Rose always said when I left the tribal center,
"Grandfather, bless. All my relations."

August

Panmuu?kak

Time of warmth

Elderhostel

The reservation is abuzz. Excitement and anticipation are palpable. Seniors are coming! The off-duty tribal police chief, dressed in a sleeveless shirt, is tending the alder fire in the pit behind the Long House. It is a warm day and smoke from the pit fills the air. Filets of salmon are split in the traditional way, down the back, secured with cross spikes and anchored to cedar stakes. The stakes are placed in the sand close enough to absorb the heat and alder smoke. Women of the tribe carry covered dishes into the community kitchen. Children practice their dramatic portrayal of Beaver Causes a Deluge. Each is to receive five dollars for the performance today. Women from the health planning group proudly display masks they are preparing to take to a presentation in Washington, D.C. The community health representative plans a grand tour of the tribal conference center and clinic, staff offices and the Long House. All clinic and administrative staff are on alert. The Long House is spit and polished ready. Soon a bus will arrive from Seattle carrying a large group of non-native senior citizens who have gathered from all over the country. The Elderhostel educational seminar will be hosted by the Cedar Bay Tribe.

The seniors arrive shortly before noon. Tribal elders greet them at the front door and they begin their tour of the reservation. Not wanting to miss any of the action, I slip downstairs and into the kitchen, grab a serving spoon and stand behind the steam table. Smoked salmon is brought in from the fire pit and scooted onto serving trays. On the large black stovetop, oysters are fried, and clam chowder heated. Fry bread, shaped by hand, sizzles on the griddle. Blackberries from nearby bushes are made into bubbly cobblers. The heads of the salmon are set aside. "Why?" I ask. "They are reserved for the elders; they are sacred."

Native elders from the reservation as well as neighboring tribes join the gathering. When all are present, we stand together for thankful prayer. Then, elders and seniors move to the head of the food line. Elders and seniors are respected. They have wisdom, years and white hair. The very best

153

is given to guests—just as in traditional potlatch. Besides salmon, oysters and clam chowder, the feast also includes Dungeness crab, elk and venison, fresh vegetable salads, potatoes, cornbread, and several desserts.

After lunch the gathering moves into the meeting room, past the table of women's story masks, to be entertained by a performance including all the children of the reservation.

Time evaporates. The tour, feast, lively discussion, interaction among elders of different cultures, viewing masks on the display table, children's performance—all begin to wind down. With parting handshakes, the visitors leave the long house and walk across the parking lot to board the bus.

While cleaning up after the guests have departed, tribal women discover the basket they left on the mask table contains three hundred dollars. The money will help the women take their masks and stories to Washington. After the guests leave the reservation, the tribe returns to mundane fare, using commodity foods to stretch a more meager food budget. As is the tradition in the potlatch, the tribe has given their very best and they have given it all.

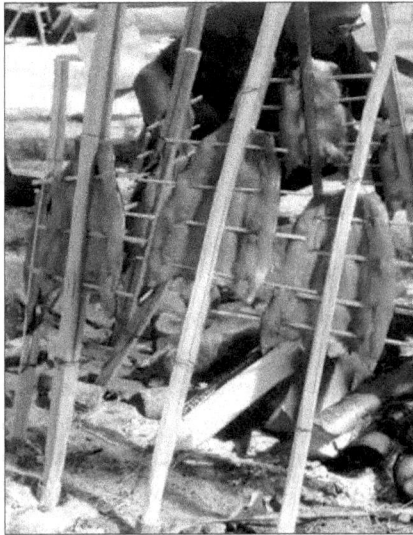

Filets of salmon are flanked, staked and placed near the alder wood fire.

At a reservation staff meeting with the tribal chairman, my mind wanders from discussion of reservation elders to my own beloved grandparents and memories of visiting them in Waverly, Ohio when I was very young.

Ya-A

Some say *Ya-A, Grandfather,* in their Prayers.
Creator.
Great Spirit.
Grandfather is an elder.
Grandfather has white hairs.
Grandfather listens.
Grandfather heals hurts.

I can see my grandfather, my Ya-A
sitting in the brown velvet chair in the living room at 414 First Avenue
on the edge of town, where around the bend meant "country"
across the road from the potato fields of the Children's Home.

I helped the kids in their chore of digging potatoes
They let me ride the work horse down the rows
Clinton Yates guiding the plow behind
unearthing tiny spuds for others to bend down, retrieve, place into their bags
complained I was riding too slowly
daydreaming from on top.

I gave horse a gentle kick
picked up speed
Clinton's feet barely touched the ground
knuckles blanched white from grip on plow handle
un-blanketed from their resting place,
potatoes flew into the air.

The velveteen arms of the chair were nubby from wear
Sitting with outstretched arms,
fingers curl wooden carved claws of the arm rest
on the floor, spitting range, the cuspidor.

Grandfather stretches long arms over the armrest
expertly clutches the cuspidor

155

aims a strong spit
nasty glob of fiber
takes a direct splat into the bowl.

Grandfather sitting in the chair,
rested his feet
on a matching brown velvet padded wrought iron stool
always covered with current newspapers.

Grandfather holds counsel from that Chair
Many come to discuss matters of importance -
Law, taxes, business, education, farming, construction, politics, medicine
he knows it all
Grandfather is very wise
He has white hairs.

He counsels me on all issues
solves my problems
doctors my wounds
treats my scraped knee
carries me piggy-back all the way into town to the doctor's office.

Those waiting in line
let Granddad take me in first
(bare footed, playing back by the barn at the Children's Home,
I had jumped from the top rung of corral fence onto a board with a rusty nail
sticking straight up
crying, holding foot in the air, I hopped home to Grandfather.)

Grandfather repaired my broken dolls.
built me a play house tucked into a corner of the family garage
complete with handmade furniture
You climbed a ladder to get into the room.

Grandfather ran for sheriff of Pike County in 1914.
Republican ticket
I know because
I came across a campaign post card with his picture on it.

The brown velvet has long since been reupholstered with brocade.
Wooden curved claws can still be seen at the end of the arm rests
padded wrought iron foot stool continues to rest the newspapers
no cuspidor nor splats of tobacco.

No potty pot on the second floor
no outhouse in back
now, modern plumbing upstairs and down
Clinton Yates has a grown family.
The potato field is covered with a school
screaming voices of running children can be heard on weekdays.

Chairman interrupts serious discourse
as his eight year old niece quietly, boldly enters the room
tension relaxes, extends his arms for the expected hug
reassurred of love, affirmed as to her presence,
niece leaves as confidently as she arrived.

In spirit, my grandfather, my Ya-A, continues to counsel
from the brown velvet chair at 414 First Avenue
he interrupts his sky counsel
whispers advice or blows on my scraped and hurting soul.

Thank you, my grandfather for watching and hugging me when I need you.
Thank you, Grandfather for listening
Thank you, Grandfather.

Ya-A

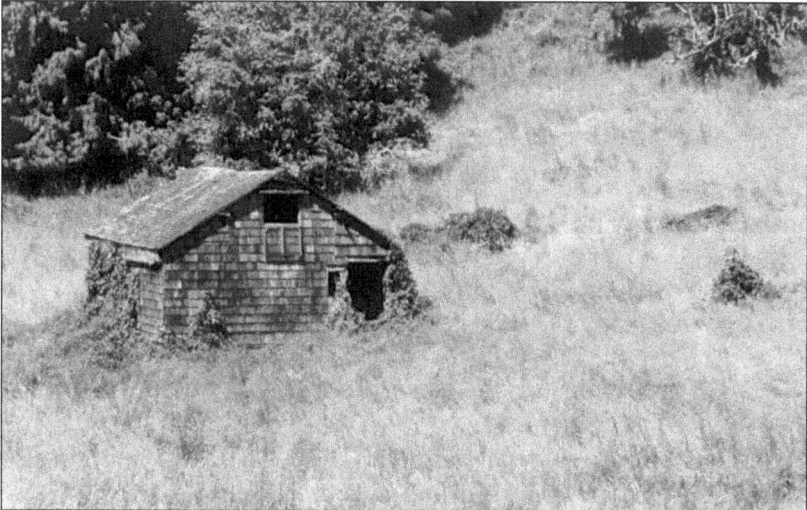

This old barn sits along the road near Willapa Bay. The sight of it connects me to the old barns of my grandparents' farm—beside Pee Pee Creek in the Pike County Valley of Southern Ohio, land of my ancestors.

September

Ts okwanpitskitlʔlak

Leaves are getting red on the vine maples

Story Mask

Animals are preparing for change, storing up for the winter ahead. On the reservation, we prepare as well. The women's planning group has decided to take their stories of loss, healing and hope to the other Washington. It is time for the annual conference of all the Robert Wood Johnson Foundation grants that are "Opening Doors: Reducing Social/Cultural Barriers to Health Care." Although the chairman represented the tribe and made the trip last year, the women prepare to go this year and share their work and their stories. They are ready to go beyond the tribal boundaries, and build on the successful groundwork of the chairman.

Eleven women come together one evening at the tribal center to make masks. The room is first purified, cleansed by smudging with sweet grass smoldering in an abalone shell. The mental health worker teaches us how to meditate and we use these techniques as plaster of Paris strips are applied to our faces. The community health worker begins with an inspirational reading of women's health and reflection. The art teacher calmly explains the process and teaches us to make the forms. Those of us who were applying the strips do so quietly and respectfully. Those to whom the strips are being applied withdraw into their own thoughts and meditations. Twenty minutes later, the strips of plaster have hardened into a mask. Calm faces then wrinkle into angry snarls and masks "pop" away from changed facial muscles. White masks are set aside to dry.

One week passes. Eleven women return to reclaim facial forms and apply paint and decoration. The masks tell stories of sorrow, loss, fear, anticipation, discovery and hope and the women await their trip to Washington, D.C. to tell their stories.

"Friends of the Tribe," an environmental group located on the other side of Willapa Bay, calls for a meeting to discuss the eco-system that caused the Cedar Bay tribal members to have a high rate of infant mortality. Friends are concerned that they are part of the same environment and considered the tribe to be a "bell weather" of the area. What happens to the tribe could happen to them. In the home of the tug boat captain, "Friends" gather—a naturopathic physician, the county public health nurse, former and retired employees of the Environmental Protection Agency, two resident Native American public health nurses—one a Chinook, the other Hurok. The community health worker and I represent the Cedar Bay Tribe.

Later that same month, the Cedar Bay Tribe invite "Friends" and area health care providers to join them for a fundraising spaghetti dinner. The fundraiser contributes $832 to send the tribal women and eleven story masks to Washington, D.C.

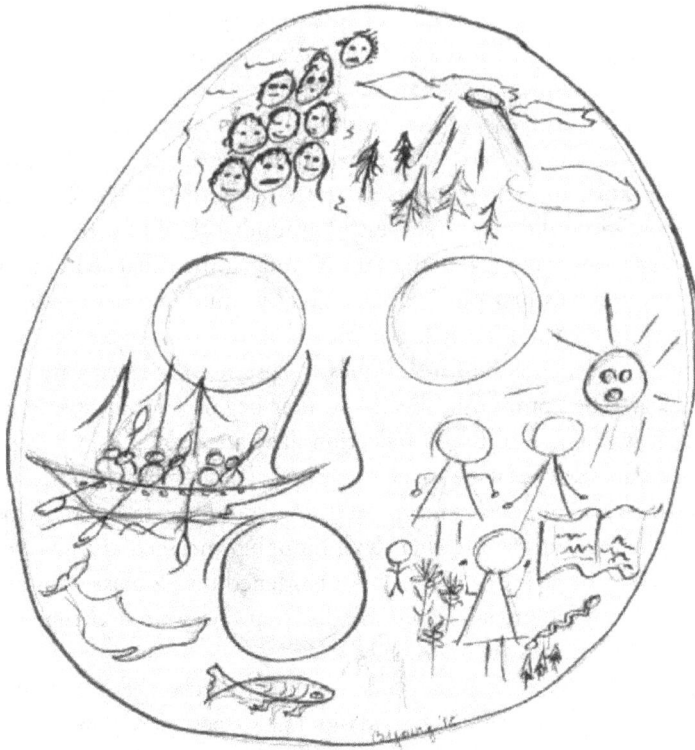

This is a sketch of my story mask, "Reflections." The sun in the east shines on my three daughters. The open book is our story and education. The snake is a symbol of health and is in touch with the earth. The salmon is vital to life in the Northwest. The canoe with paddlers represents the tribe. The whale passes not far off shore on its annual migration. The choir represents ancestors. Mt. Rainier is a retreat for hiking and cross-country skiing.

160

October

Pan?silpaulos

Time of autumn

Trip to Washington, D.C.

Autumn in D.C. is unlike the misty Pacific Northwest. There is crispness in the air. Colored crunchy leaves are falling from the trees, a memory of summer's shade and harbinger of the coming winter. From Washington state to Washington, D.C. we go, from Willapa Bay to the Chesapeake Bay.

We are tired when we arrive at DuPont Circle and check into the hotel, but we are not too tired to head to the streets and negotiate the strangely laid out city. Streets are spokes of a wheel. This is not the same as on the reservation where the medicine wheel held everything in calm balance and where the center of the wheel is the grounding of self.

Having lived in nearby Richmond, Virginia and being somewhat familiar with the city, I wanted to show them everything. I begin the tour: "Here is the White House, right here! Soon we will be on the Mall and see the Smithsonian Institute Buildings—The American History Museum, the National Gallery of Art, the Hirshhorn, the Washington Monument. Do you know the architect, I. M. Pei? He designed an incredible razor-sharp edge to the building of the east wing of the National Gallery of Art where Calder mobiles hang in the lobby atrium! We can also walk to the Lincoln Memorial." The women scarcely have time to breathe or respond.

I'm so absorbed in my excitement that I forget to listen to their feelings. I ignore their silence. The early morning drive to the airport on the west coast, the flight across the country and now the hustle of the eastern capitol city is more than enough for one day. Our spirits are confused, disoriented and disconnected. I am feeling the political pace of the city. They, instead, feel its power, oppression and are not emotionally separated from the west coast reservation. We end the tour and return to the hotel.

The following day the women unpack the carefully carried, bubble-wrapped masks, and display them on two tables in the exhibit room of the conference we are attending. Hard copies of written stories are laid beside each mask.

We present our formal report to the administrative staff of our grant and twenty-one other grant participants like ourselves. The tribal women of the Cedar Bay sit front and center. They sit tall and visible to all who are attending the meeting. We are scheduled to present our project report late in the afternoon. As coordinator of "The Return to Health" project of the Cedar Bay Indian Tribe, I sit on a panel with three other grant project leaders. When it is time to speak, the tribal health coordinator comes forward, the room lights dim and the first slide is projected, sharing the women's stories, their loss and their struggle of survival.

When the session ends, I look for approval from the three tribal women sitting in the front row. They come forward and hug me, letting me know I have done well. The future of the grant is no longer dependent upon my presentation.

I stand back and let the tribal women receive hugs from others who come forward to recognize their work: Hispanic women from inner-Chicago, black women from the south, Native Americans from the Southwest. Tears of understanding and love come from women of color from all parts of the nation. "We understand. We see your stories in the masks." Absent were understanding hugs from white women.

Washington is exhilarating. However, it is not the reservation. We pack our bags and walk through the sculpture gardens on the ellipse. We buy souvenir t-shirts from the open stalls on the Mall. We look with awe toward the Capitol Building and wave in the opposite direction to the Washington Monument. Now, I am in tune with the women. The sun is shining and we laugh. We continue our tour. Although we are exhausted, there is a spring in our step as we direct our path home.

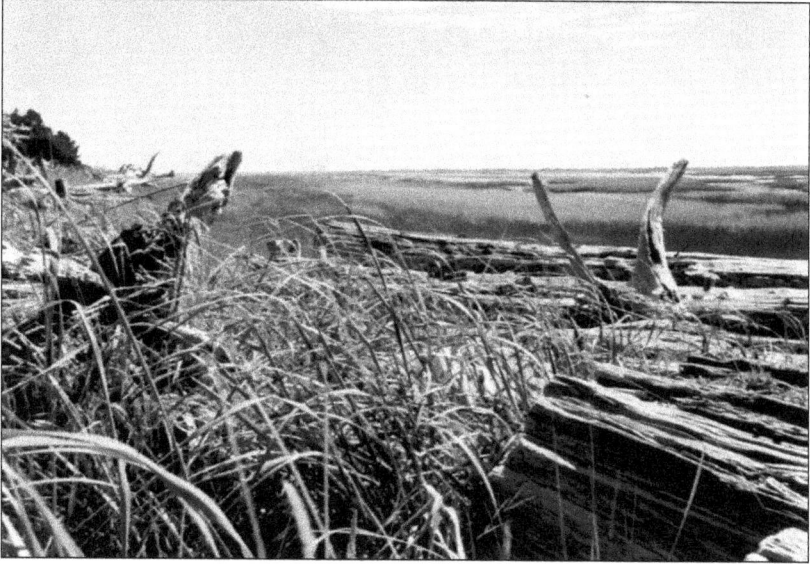

From the congested city of Washington, to the forests and isolation of the tidewaters. From east to west, from Atlantic to Pacific, from Chesapeake to the Willapa. We fly over four mountain ranges—the Appalachians, the Ozarks, the Rockies, and the Cascades. We cross three time zones. We head west. We are going home. I often have lunch at this spot, near the tribal center, on the mud flats and tidewaters of Willapa Bay.

Strategies in Communication

We settle back into our work and routine. I have not received official word whether grant monies will be extended into the next year. Perhaps there is still a chance to communicate about our work. I plan to attend a conference of grant administrators for forty Robert Wood Johnson Foundation grant programs. Others might have insight into more effective lines of communication between project and funder. There is no grant money left for my travel, but the chairman allows the time away for me to attend. How I get to San Francisco for the conference is entirely up to me. A flight to San Jose, Cal Train and city buses and staying with high school friends near the city makes it all work out.

Once at the conference, I find a seat, listen carefully, and speak up on issues such as: the ability to communicate between east coast funder and west coast Indian reservation; setting project priorities; what happens when the recipients who are to guide the grant project disagree with priorities set by the funder; "time" definitions and requirements between cultures; how to deal with power and control of grant monies; how to listen to the concerns of others—both funder and recipient. It is a stimulating discussion and soon it is time for lunch.

I am up early the next day. My friend's daughter drives me into the city, saving valuable time. The conference is over at noon. I shop in Chinatown, buy a canvas bag for my accumulated papers and gifts and board the bus for the Cal Train station. I ride to San Jose, then catch a bus to the airport and fly home.

Back in Seattle after midnight—my car is covered with soggy leaves from a heavy rain. I discover that I have left my raincoat, with the car keys in the pocket, hanging in my friend's closet in sunny Palo Alto. I pay a locksmith to open my car and craft a new key so that I may drive in the night back home.

The conference in San Francisco was called Strategies in Communication. As I study the petroglyphs of the Columbia River Gorge at Vantage, Washington, I ponder what the first peoples were communicating to us through their drawings and recordings in stone.

◆ ◆ ◆ ◆ ◆

It is Dad's weekend at Washington State University in Pullman. Near the Idaho border and in the middle of the Palouse, golden wheat fields of eastern Washington welcome the dads to the university, a city within a city. Since football is not a priority for daughter Susan, I spend time with her in the microbiology labs. We begin our day feeding and weighing the lab rats in the science wing of the veterinary school. Susan is involved in a study of brain cancer caused by excess estrogen.

On my way home I stop at Ginkgo Petrified Forest State Park. Inside the stone park center, I watch the informational movie which shows that this was once a ginkgo forested area. A professor in the 1940's directed his anthropology class to dig for fossils and found petrified wood, as the professor had predicted. A ginkgo forest in what is now desert!

I purchase a tiny ginkgo seedling and prepare to leave. But first, one last look at the mighty and beautiful Columbia River before I travel west over Snoqualmie Pass. I follow a stone walkway around the building to the edge of the cliff. Overlooking the water is a cascade of petroglyph rock carvings, a strategy of communication of people who once lived in this area.

The petroglyths show a family—two parents and a child between them—touching. The parents have headdresses, or were they halos? The sun is carved on a rock above the others. A squiggly line might be a crooked path or switchbacks we take along the way. Four-legged running animals are distinct in the rock. One figure holds hands with another. Some four-leggeds have long horns. Four circles, one within the other, are highlighted by their light and dark contrast. I sense continuity of life. I retrace the steps to my car, belt in the tiny seedling and drive west.

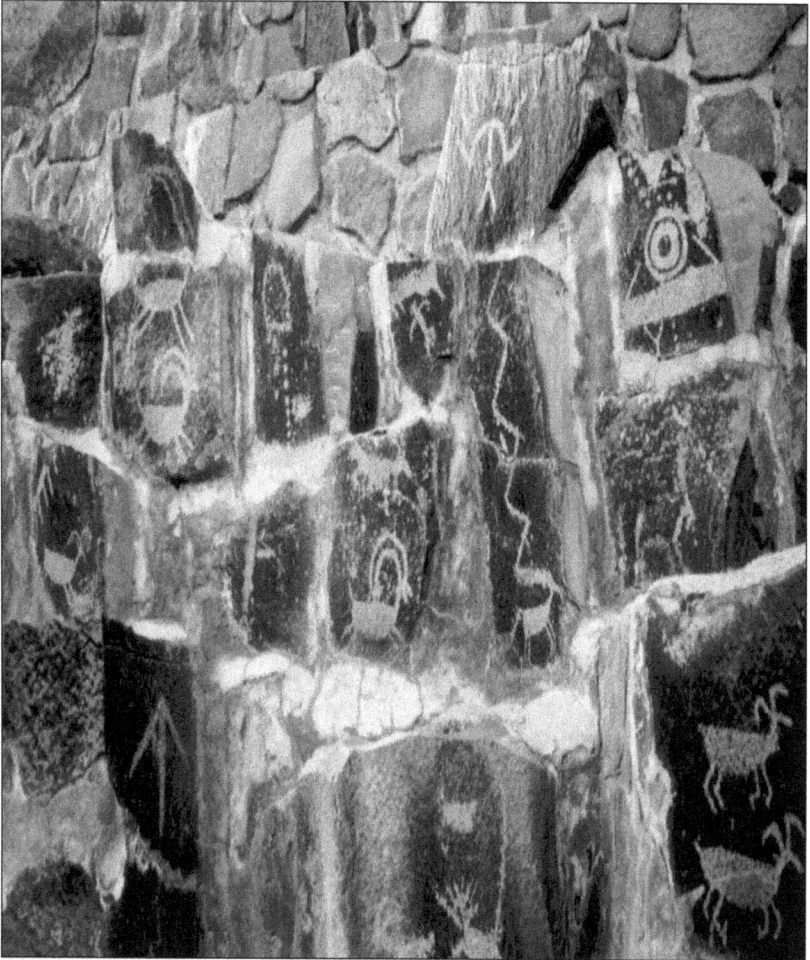

Barbara M. Young

These petroglyphs were salvaged from lower banks of the Columbia River before the construction of the Bonneville Dam. When the decision was made to dam the Columbia River for irrigation and recreation, these were saved by moving to an elevated cliff at Vantage, Washington.

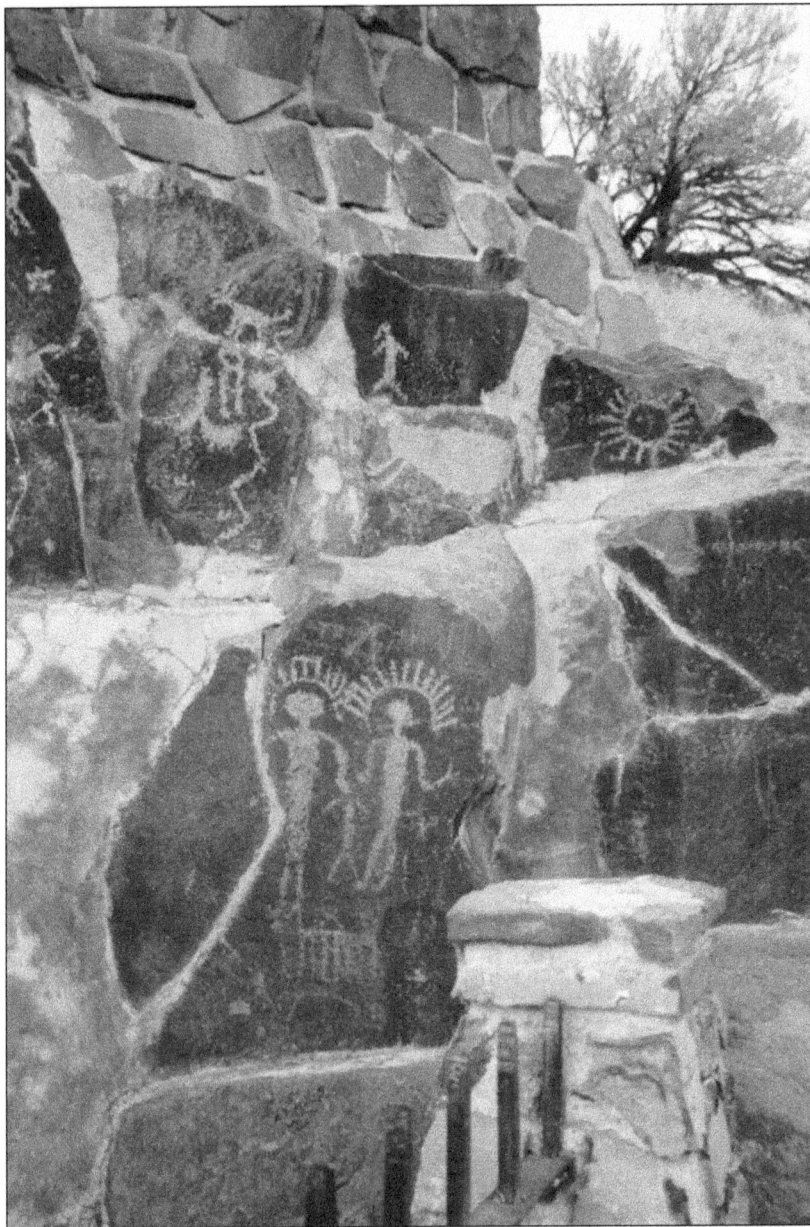

Barbara M. Young

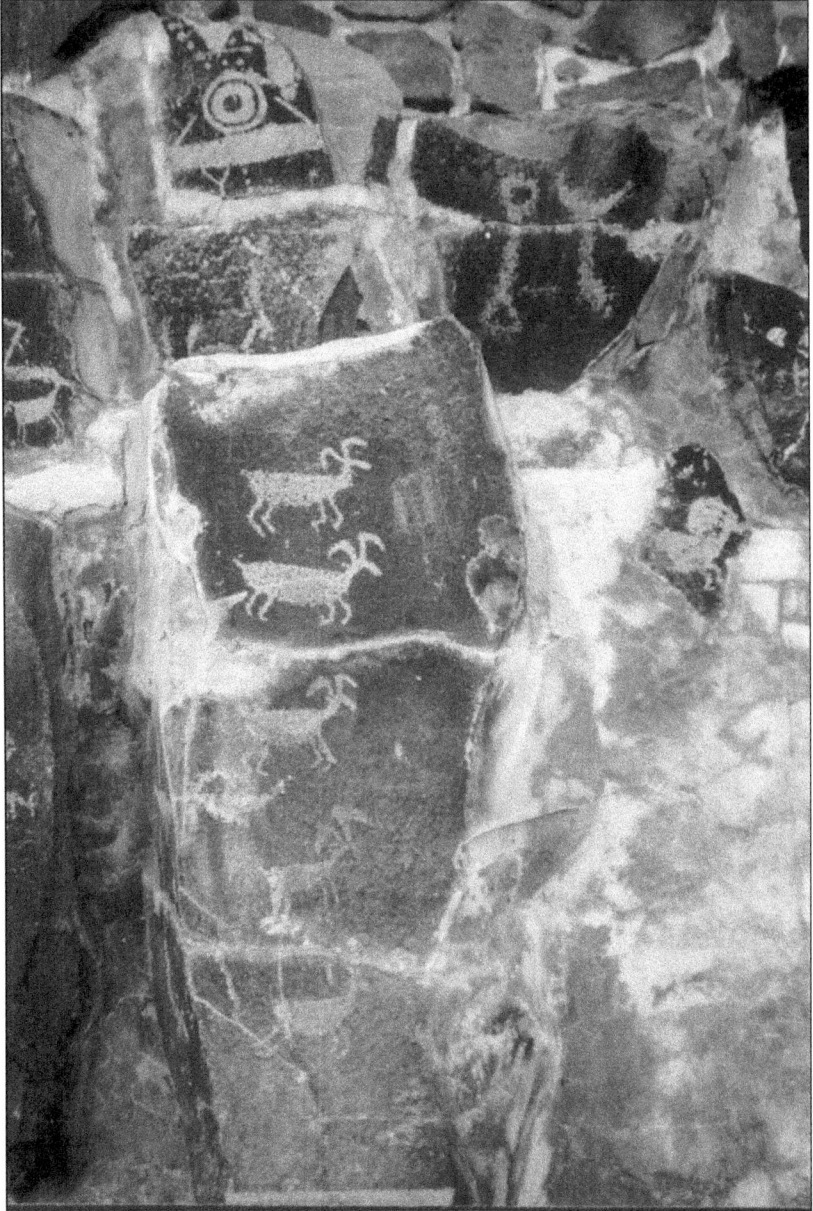

Barbara M. Young

November

Panitpuhtuhkstista

Time when the clouds are covering

The Public Health Meeting

It is November and time to attend the annual meeting of the American Public Health Association in New York City. The theme is Empowering the Disadvantaged—Social Justice in Public Health. My sister gives me her frequent flyer coupon. My brother will put me up in New Jersey. Conference registration is $250 and my year's membership to the APHA is $100. If I skip the nurse's luncheon, dress for walking, and take the subways, I can financially make the trip and have the networking and contacts. The chairman gives me permission for a week's leave of absence.

The conference is electrifying. The first day begins with a session by the Native American/Alaskan Native and Native Hawaiian caucus. Dr. June Strickland of the University of Washington, a Native American nursing professor, presents her research with the Nooksack tribe. Her study of pain is applicable to the pain and grief on the Cedar Bay reservation.

The next day, I hop the A Train to Harlem Hospital to learn how the tuberculosis program is dramatically reducing the number of cases in an epidemic of multiple-drug resistant tuberculosis. After the session, I leave the hospital and see the streets of Harlem come alive with light and music.

There is a nurses' gathering at the Henry Street Settlement House, the birthplace of public health nursing founded by Lillian Wald in 1893. During a class in home nursing, Lillian was called from the classroom by a small child asking her to visit her sick mother. She followed the child through the streets of the Lower East Side to a cluttered staircase which they climbed to the third floor. In the darkened apartment, the mother was two days post-delivery. Her husband, attentive and proud, needed directions on how to help his wife. Lillian sent the father for fish to make soup. She, meanwhile, helped bathe the new mother and taught care of the newborn. Lillian came to recognize the fierce pride of the people and the need for nursing care to reach into the community. Lillian became a community activist for new immigrants, and leaned on her merchant friends for money to open the Henry Street Settlement House. Lillian asked political friends, including President Woodrow Wilson, for help in establishing health policies that addressed public health in the tenements.

Early public health nurses trained at Henry Street clinic in the program that Wald founded. The nurses lived—up to ninety-five at a time—in the small quarters on the upper floors of the house. They taught young immigrant mothers home nursing skills and how to care for themselves and their families. "The nurses empowered the young mothers," our current day host says. Empowerment is not a modern idea. Lillian, over one hundred years ago, preached these ideas. We exit the original building of the Henry Street settlement and walk the cobblestone street to the new theater where neighborhood children participate in expressive drama. In addition to the theater, the new building also houses a day care center where recently arrived immigrant children are exposed to the new language and culture surrounded by relaxed, caring teachers and colorful books and toys.

Impressed by the continuation of Lillian Wald's work and its importance to those recently arrived, our tiny group of four nurses exits and walks toward Mulberry Street for lunch. The few trees we pass are beautiful and strong, surviving the traffic and brick and new populations. Each tree receives sufficient sunshine, water and nourishment, which reminds us of how we need each other to survive.

The Annual Meeting of Public Health is over. I have walked the same cobblestone street as Lillian Wald; I have networked with my colleagues. Nursing Professor Janet and I decide it is time to enjoy the Big Apple. Enough of business; it is time for play.

Janet notices a free concert at Lincoln Center with Julliard students performing. The concert is in progress, so we slip into a back row: A Mozart cello and piano concerto is a contrast to the hurried streets and intense conference we just left. Later, Janet walks me to the Port Authority where I will take a bus to Roseland, New Jersey, where my brother Jerry meets my bus at 12:30 a.m. When I recount the intense day, Jerry reminds me of our musical New York relatives. An uncle trained at Julliard and was a church organist. Aunt Lois was a piano teacher who studied at the Toronto Conservatory. The family story is that Aunt Lois' grand piano had to be lifted by crane into her fifth floor Long Island apartment where she taught for many years. Because I first visited New York when I was twelve, I am connected to this city as surely as I am connected to the tidewaters of the Pacific Coast.

◆ ◆ ◆ ◆ ◆

The next morning after a cup of strong east coast coffee (Seattle doesn't hold the patent on good coffee), Jerry and I begin the methodical and yearly fall ritual of leaf raking. Crisp colorful leaves of all varieties are raked onto large tarps to be pulled either to the street for city pick-up or to the woods in the lot next to the house. I had forgotten the pleasure and the fall smells of eastern trees. Maples. Oaks. Cottonwoods. Birch. The crunch as I rake releases husky, musky, dusty earthy smells I can taste. The city leaf machine sucks up the leaves at the curb, but the piles in the woods are up for grabs. As I did fifty years before, I take a running dive into the gathered pile and am quickly buried in the colorful, glorious, crackly crunch of autumn leaves. The smell that engulfs me reminds me of the two grand-mother maples that occupied the entire space of our front yard in Dayton and also provided leaf piles for the entire block of kids to enjoy.

The zillion leaves now in my brother's New Jersey woods remind me of grandmother's feather bed in southern Ohio. Lying there, I look up into the clear blue sky beyond the leafless branches standing as protective sentinels to my private fall world.

It is time to catch my flight from Newark and return to the west coast and the reservation, trading musky autumn deciduous groves for piney evergreen forests; honking taxis and commuter buses for calm clam digging on isolated shores and tidewaters. Time to take the lessons learned at Henry Street Settlement and Harlem Hospital to the Native American Long House. Lillian Wald would have understood returning to the Indian community and applying lessons of advocacy for environmental health. She would have approved of local political leadership in determining health policy, empowering the people who would strengthen the family, the very basis of community health. I am going home.

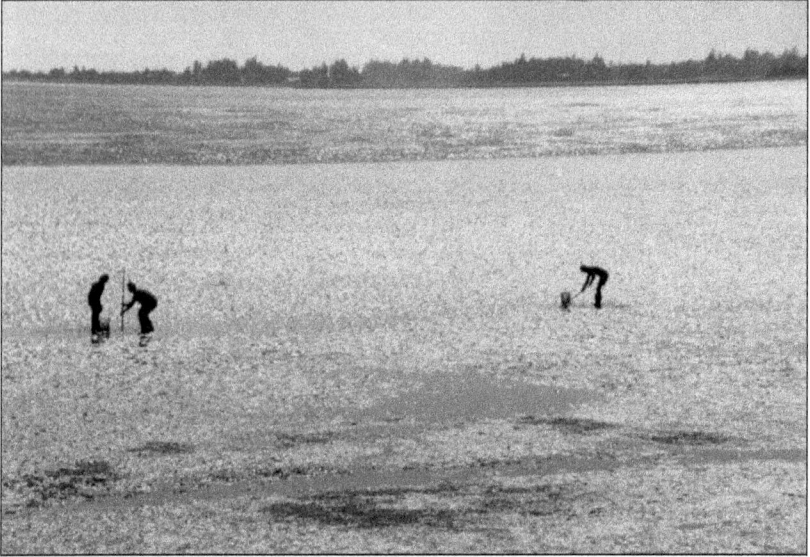

Clam digging on the mud flats and tidewaters of Willapa Bay.

Funeral Mass

LeAnn was the tribal elder fighting cancer while I was working on the reservation. Although the disease—and her treatment—sapped nearly every ounce of her strength, she continued to ask questions about her care. She remained in charge. She undertook each recommended therapy and experimental test so that the disease had every chance for remission. Through it all, she maintained a sense of humor that sustained her mother and cousin—her main caregivers— as well as the nursing and medical staff. She used her remaining time to teach us all what it was like to be a cancer patient with a terminal illness. She taught us about healing and wellness. She taught us about dying. She taught us about life.

Today, two hundred mourners file into the church. My daughter Susan accompanies me to the memorial service. She has helped me host LeAnn's mother, Elenna, her Aunt Irene, and her friend Edith at our home during hospital stays for chemotherapy. The funeral service is held in the Catholic Church in town. The priest begins by calling the congregation to prayer, swinging a brass incense burner on a long chain, back and forth. He speaks in Latin. Organ music accompanies hymns. The congregation is invited to take communion, the ceremonial sacrament of the Last Supper, symbols of forgiveness and resurrected life. The priest completes his part of the service with prayer and sits down in the first pew.

A drummer friend of LeAnn, accompanied by his wife and Edith, begins to beat softly on drums, again calling the gathered to prayer. A Native American spiritual leader walks forward to the space vacated by the priest. In consideration of non-native mourners, he briefly explains his ritual, then begins to sing the opening prayer in his own tribal language. In his prayer, he calls the gathered mourners to join him in gratitude to The Great Spirit for the forests and the animals and all that walk, fly and crawl upon Mother Earth. The spiritual leader holds an abalone shell in which sage is smoldering, not unlike the incense burner of the Catholic priest. He walks down the aisle and wafts smoke with a feather fan. He eulogizes

LeAnn's life and speaks of the significance of the gathering. Then, drummers and chanters sing to LeAnn's spirit.

After the service, we walk to the social hall for a feast of celebration. There are salads and veggie trays, pies, cakes, chips and dip. There is salmon and berry cobbler. Susan studies the posters on the walls that depict the forty years of LeAnn's life. I had known LeAnn for a brief two years, but in that time I learned much from her. In the end she taught us all how to die with dignity, grace and love. LeAnn is buried not far from the Catholic Church where we celebrated her life.

◆ ◆ ◆ ◆ ◆

For the canoe people of the Columbia River area, burial was a different, sacred rite of passage. The dead were ceremoniously placed in their canoes with all of the tools that they would need in the next life, including beads of stone and glass, elk teeth and coins, arrowheads, knives, tomahawks and flintlock guns. Women were buried with their favorite basket, beads and other ornaments important to them. The bodies were covered with woven mats and blankets. The canoes were set in the branches of fir and spruce, or paddled down river to the Isle of the Dead on the Columbia River. It was a sacred burial ground recognized and used by all tribes in the area. Some of the families built cedar shelters within which their deceased rested. Others elevated the burial canoe on rocks. Holes were drilled into the canoe to allow for water drainage as well as to make them unusable for the living. After a year, bones were collected by family members and buried with the ancestral bones in family or tribal graves. When whites overran the area, Indian sacred burial grounds were desecrated. Canoes, tools, mats, baskets and knives were stolen. Thieves did not respect the spirits.

Victor Trevitt was a white saloon owner, gambler and politician from the Dalles, Oregon, who stipulated he was to be buried among the Indians on the Isle of the Dead. Victor wrote that the white man was treacherous; his own chances of entering heaven were better with a native group of Indians. He thought that St. Peter might overlook him and allow him to enter heaven if he were among a group of honest people. On a cold February day, a steamer carried the body and marker of Victor Trevitt to burial island where he was laid to rest.

When tribes heard that Trevitt had violated their sacred burial grounds, they canoed to the island at night and removed the blanket wrapped forms and bones of their ancestors and took them to another place. The ground was no longer sacred. Never again would the Natives use the island for burial. The canoes and cedar lodges have long since washed away. Bonneville Dam flooded much of the island. Only the tomb of Victor Trevitt can still be seen from the Oregon side of the river. Trevitt is alone.

❖ ❖ ❖ ❖ ❖

My parents are buried in the Masonic section of the Dayton Memorial Gardens according to the secret rituals of the Masonic order. I never knew my father's sacred rituals, but I respected them and honored his belief. My father's parents, whom I never knew, are buried in a mausoleum in Ontario, Canada. My mother's parents and grandparents and great grandparents and other relatives are buried in the Union Cemetery in Waverly, Ohio, about an hour's drive north of the Ohio River. I had thought to bury with my mother a kitchen implement or something fun for her afterlife—a deck of cards for the bridge games she so loved with her friends. My sister disapproved and instead, slipped into the coffin a broach our father had given our mother when they were both young and in love. I still have the deck of cards. They have never been played.

❖ ❖ ❖ ❖ ❖

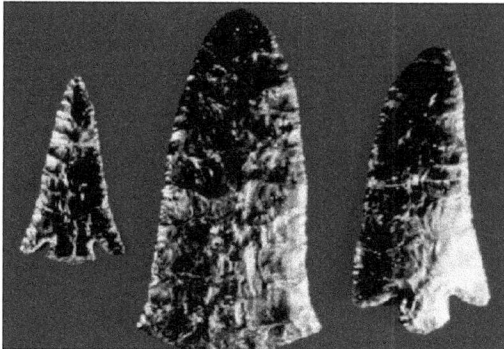

This picture of arrowheads was taken from a slide sold at Mound City, near Chillicothe, Ohio. My siblings and I collected arrowheads on our hikes along creek beds and ditches near the town of Waverly where my grandparents lived. These finds were relinquished to my grandfather who in turn sent them to the Ohio Historical Society.

A sacred Indian site of the Missippippi Valley People is Serpent Mound in Adams County, Ohio. It is believed that this site, built to face the solstice, is not for burial but for ceremony and ritual. It was constructed on a hill top above Brush Creek, discovered by anthropologists in the 1800s and saved from the farmer's plow when it was designated a state historical park.

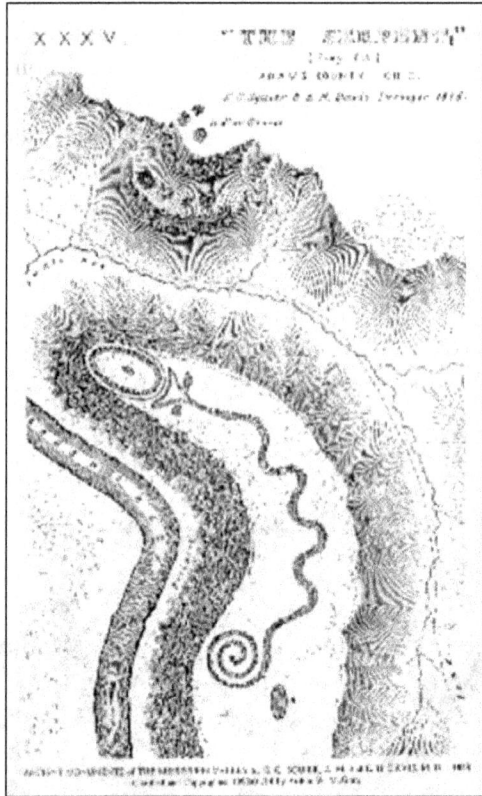

This 1846 aerial sketch by E .G. Squire and E. H. Davis Surveyors, titled "The Serpent," depicts the serpent ready to engulf an egg, and was the documentation needed to save the area as a state monument.

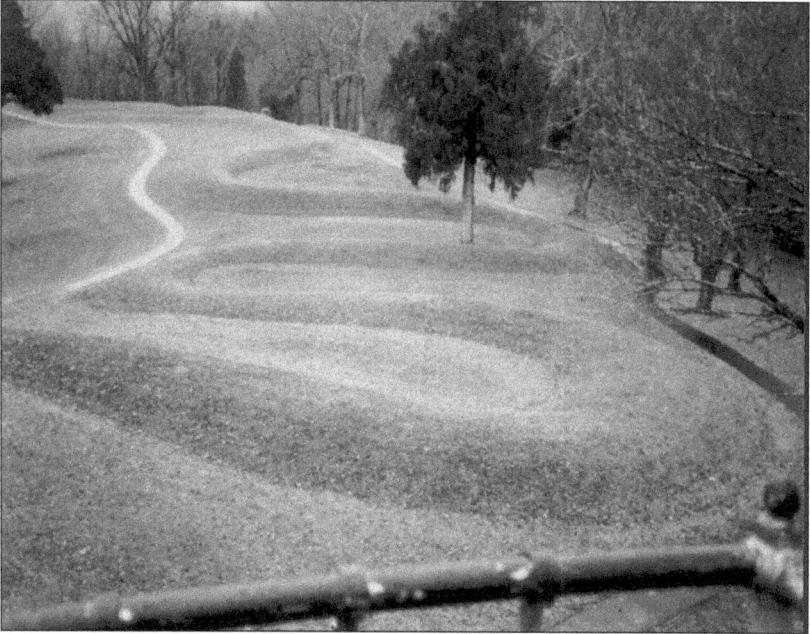

Barbara M. Young

Serpent Mound is now a state park surrounded by cornfields, country and gentle woods.

Indian Sacred Burial Mounds and Ancient Clan Cairns

I was four years old when my parents took me to visit Serpent Mound. Climbing the steps of the lookout tower over tree top level seemed steep and difficult. From the wooden platform, I looked down and over a vast stretch of land into which had been built, with earth, a long and curvy serpent. The serpent was about to swallow a large egg—many times its size—and the serpent itself was many times my height. My mother said that people lived thousands of years ago here in the southern Ohio Valley. Historians do not know what the mounds contain, but we knew this site was sacred. Even at age four, I knew to respect this place.

Serpent Mound is one example of the construction and architecture of the Mound Builders. Archeologists of the 1930s and 40s excavated burial mounds at Mound City, three miles north of Chillicothe, Ohio. They found what was later described as burial chambers that contained the bones of clans of earlier cultures.

> The graves were carefully constructed with layers of gravel and pebbles and equipped with ornamental pots, effigy pipes, elk and bear teeth, and obsidian points. One mound within a complex contained a quantity of fossil mammoth or mastodon bones. Some mounds contained various ornaments of copper and shell, stone pipes and finely crafted pottery vessels. It was believed that the burial house, which was built to house the body, was eventually destroyed. Another mound was constructed over the site. This particular group of mounds in Chillicothe is believed to have been built by the Mound Builders group. One name given to these people is Hopewell Indians, because the mound city site was originally discovered on a farm owned by a Mr. Hopewell. The other culture in this area is the Adena. The archeologists believe that the later Indian culture came into the same area and used the already existing burial mounds to bury their dead. *(Silverberg, 1970)*

It was an example of one culture over another.

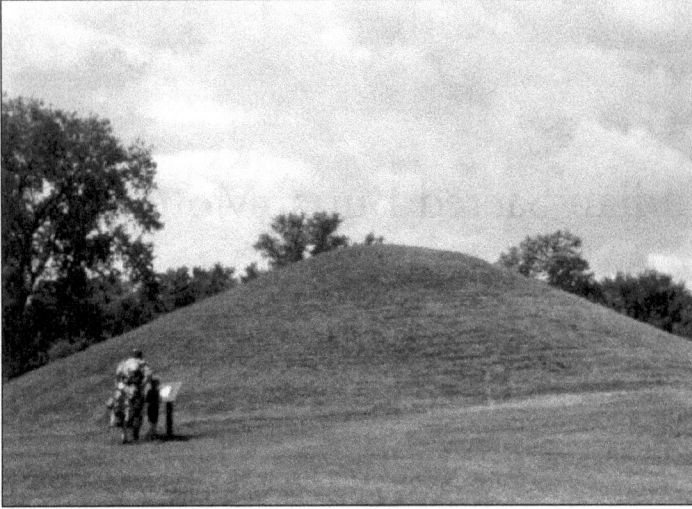

Barbara M. Young

This photo was taken at Mound City in Chillicothe, Ohio. The mound is one of twenty-three in what was known as a city.

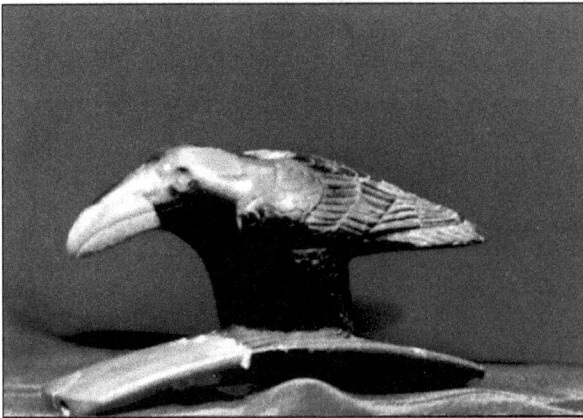

This picture was taken from a slide sold at Mound City, Chillicothe. The raven pipe was excavated from a burial mound of the Hopewell or Adena cultures in Ohio. The raven is a legendary character in the stories of the Pacific Northwest Coastal Indians, often a trickster and always teaching important life lessons.

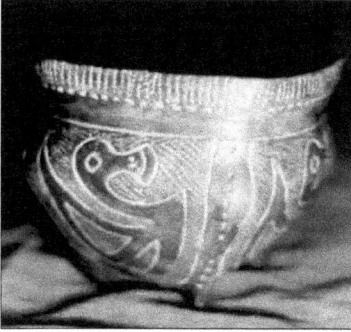

The photo is a Duck Pot credited to the peoples of the Ohio and Mississippi Valleys. In a college art class, I remember studying this design and replicating it as my own clay bowl.

Several years ago, I traveled to Glasgow, Scotland, where my daughter Katherine was in her junior year abroad. Daughter Carolyn Sue and her husband met me in Glasgow and we left early the next morning for the Highlands of Scotland and the Isle of Skye. It was March and bitterly cold. Snow covered the ground and a biting wind accompanied us for our drive north. Afternoon tea warmed us. In these lands, we were being connected to a sense of ancestry and to a Celtic culture from which our great-great-great grandparents descended.

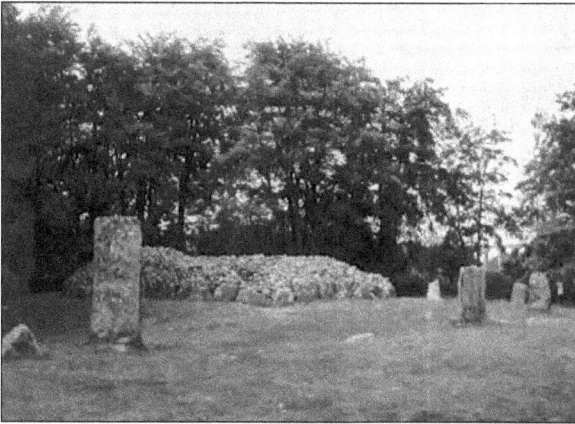

The burial mound, Clava Cairns, of the ancient Celts in the Scottish Highlands was constructed on sacred ground surrounded by guardian stone sentries. The cairn was nearby the Battlefield of Culloden. On Culloden Field Bonnie Prince Charlie and the Duke of Chamberlain met in a final battle that destroyed the Scottish clan life and determined English rule.

When the Vikings invaded and discovered the ancient Celtic gravesites, they buried their own within. The Vikings wrote on the Celtic graves, adding names on signs outside the gravesite. The two cultures lie buried together.

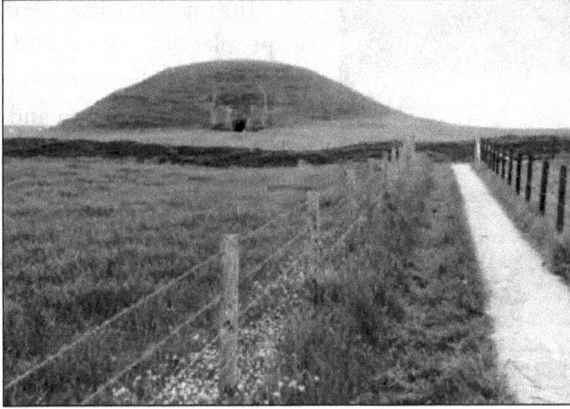

This cairn is Maes Howe on Orkney Island, north of Scotland. The small door is a passageway, lit only during sunset on the winter solstice.

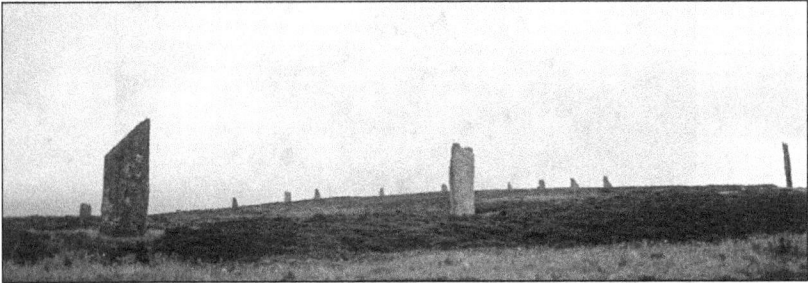

This circle of stones, some three times the height of a tall man and covering a half-mile, is the Ring of Brodgar, built on a high hill overlooking the water. It is in the Orkney Islands, on two small lakes in sight of the Atlantic Ocean and the North Sea. The Ring of Brodgar is within sight of Maes Howe.

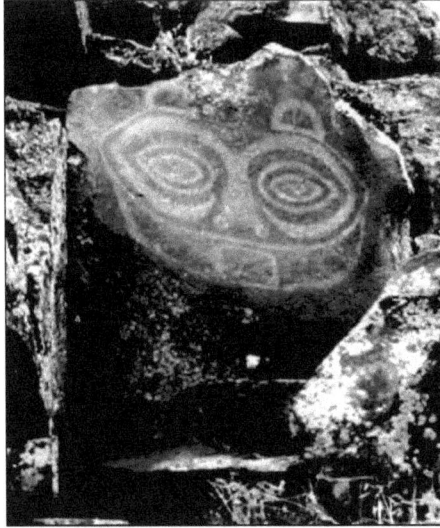

Daughter Katherine and I visited the petroglyph–pictograph, *Tsgaglalia*, She-Who-Watches. A park ranger guided us among the high rock-outfacing, remnant of a volcanic flow millions of years ago. He pointed out petroglyphs, and in one place we saw the insignia of an Air Force captain who left his initials near the ancient painting—one culture placing its signs over another. Rounding the last bend we saw the watchful eyes of Tsgaglalia. The legend is that she protected her people from communicable diseases. Coyote wanted her to give up the leadership of the tribe and give it to a male leader. Tsgaglalia had been a good leader and did not want to be tricked by Coyote. Because she did not do as Coyote demanded, Tsgaglalia, the Wishram chief, was transformed from human to rock. As leader and guardian of her people, she continues to exercise her authority.

December

Panklich

Time of darkness

Buddies

To my co-worker Edith George,

We have not learned how to communicate—
She and I;
Too many social and cultural barriers to defend
'Til we can see ... eye to eye—
History ... Family ... Home—

She lives by the shoal water.
I, in the city, eighty miles away.
She has a tall Totem outside her house
And a Northwest Owl family clan crest by her door.
By my door is a flower box
In which my Norwegian friend will plant spring bulbs.
The MacGregor crest I claim, My Race is Royal, comes from the highlands
of Scotland.

She angrily thrashes out at me;
She who guards carefully the Tribe's treasures,
For I am treading on years of loss.
She lost a son in a fishing accident on the Columbia.
I lost a grandson to adoption in Texas.
Her Tribe does not want to chance another loss
Due to my beautiful vision of health ....

She remains within the Tribe to lead the program—
Community Participation for Health.
I leave to teach students in another city—
Nursing Care with Families in the Community.
Risk.
Take no risk.
Step forward.
Slip back.

The Tree Is Medicine

At a recent Indian meeting of Women and Girls
in a forested boy scout camp
half way between her house and mine,
She approaches me
puts her arms around my shoulders
silently hugs me
examining my face
stepping back to see me,
she says.

Circle of Life

What IS the answer to high infant mortality at the Cedar Bay?

A summary of possible causes

Lunchtime, and I take a break from writing. Herb Maller gives me his bayside home so that I might have privacy to write while he winters in Yuma. From the cupboard I select a can of red sockeye salmon with a Friday Harbor label, a fishing boat in front of two snow-peaked mountains. Friday Harbor is further up the Washington coast on San Juan Island. Grabbing a big mug for tea, I see enameled on the side of the mug these words, "Schedule for Today."

9:00	Get a million dollars
10:00	Take over company
11:00	Make those who ignored you crawl
12:00	Lunch in Jamaica
1:00	Buy Jamaica
2:00	Close deal for movie on your life
3:00	Accept leading role in that movie
4:00	Advise the President
5:00	Accept award for being best person ever

Strange how far away those words are, how unattached to the real world. I contemplate and write. It's only a mug on the shelf that the manufacturer thought clever and funny.

Heating water in the mug, I reuse a well-worn tea bag, slice a mini-baguette and pad it with butter. Placing the can of salmon and the bread into a blue plastic fish-shaped bowl, I collect the mug and head to the picnic table on the deck.

The tide is coming in. Waves provide a rhythm, a continuous melody to the otherwise silent beachfront. Nothing else seems to be moving. Across the bay in the tiny village of Nahcotta behind the cannery and mountains of oyster shells, Ellen and Phil Mason tend to spring perennials, snugly planting seeds in the soil and knowing sunshine will soon replace the storms. The fake red geraniums in the flower boxes on Herb's deck are in bright contrast to the muted blues of the water, sky, distant hill and Mason's peninsula. Theirs is a thin thread of light blue horizon between a lighter blue-clouded sky and the gray-blue of incoming currents.

When I tell people of my work at Cedar Bay, they continue to ask, "What is the reason for the high rate of infant mortality?" I know they harbor their own theories and would like those theories affirmed. The high rate of infant mortality of the Cedar Bay, well documented in studies in 1992, is a tragic and dramatic reality. We, in the dominant culture, want to place blame. We want it fixed. We certainly do not want to engage in anything like it—loss, pain, suffering. The high rate of infant mortality in this tiny community could be a symbol of our own inadequacies, our in-completeness and our failure to grow in wisdom. Read my biases. We can no longer say to a small tribe, a nation on the edge, struggling for survival, that if you (the tribe) had only:

- not eaten modern foods laden with chemical preparation, interrupt-ing ancient ways of gathering

- not been poor and small

- not ingested alcohol or chemical substances

- not eaten the traditional salmon from contaminated streams (since we chose to clear cut the forests to supply our paper demands)

- not accessed western medical practices (because native medicine peo-ple are gone)

- been better assimilated into the dominant society and accepting of our contemporary ways (instead of confining yourselves to reserved lands and clinging to ancient cultures, language, dance, and medicine)

- lived longer to teach us your wisdom (native elders die years sooner than the dominant culture elderly)

The grave markers of the infants of Cedar Bay speak to all of us. They are our children as well as theirs. We cry, "It takes a village." We have not come together as a village or community to speak up for the existing con-ditions that allow our children to die. This tribe on the brink of non-exis-tence, on land that is sliding into the sea, is a symbol of our own chances for survival. "We can only know the future in the laughter of healthy chil-dren." (Dame Whina Cooper, Maori Kuia, elder. Schaef, A.W., *Native Wisdom for White Minds*)

What **is** the reason for the high infant mortality rate at the Cedar Bay?

Lack of access to care? Could be. It took over a year to find a dedicated medical doctor to commit to serving at the tribal clinic. It also took the women a long time to have the confidence to communicate adequately with the western trained medical providers.

Environmental toxins? Would the stories of thousands of dead Dungeness crabs strewn along the beach or a flock of birds lying dead on the shore give a clue to environmental poisons?

Chemical substance abuse? Michael Dorris in *The Broken Cord* describes rearing a child with fetal alcohol syndrome, the heartache that can result from maternal alcoholism. Could this also be a concern on this reservation?

Poverty? I was paid by a funding grant and hired because I had a master's degree. My colleague had a similar job description. She did not have academic credentials, was a tribal elder, member of the Council, knew the history of the grief and loss, and knew the tribal members. She had the "inside information." I had the "outside information." Her salary was half of mine. "That's the salary on the reservation," she said.

Ignorance? Perhaps, if the tribe remained isolated and remote, the ills of the larger dominant society would not affect them, but in this global community, it is not possible to remain protected from disease and ill behavior. The Chinook once inhabited the area from the Columbia River to the Chehalis River to the Pacific Coast. When smallpox, measles and syphilis were introduced, their numbers went from 160,000 to 1600. They lost future generations, medicine people and elders. Now they participate in county health assessment under the state Public Health Improvement Plan. They collaborate with the Pacific County Health Department. They invite speakers to discuss diabetes. Young women ask questions concerning gestational diabetes. They seek information about heart disease, adding exercise and healthy eating to their routines; add nutritional lessons for children being tutored after school; hire a mental health worker to meet with their children and a native storyteller to discuss family issues; and invite an acting group to dramatize delicate family relationships. They seek the balance of the ancient wisdom in the medicine wheel.

Soul loss? Spirit sickness? When I first arrived, I sensed hopelessness. The tribal community was in mourning. Their grief was compounded by the loss of culture, land, life style and traditional diet. Their baskets had been sold to white dealers and were absent from the reservation.

Lack of traditional diet? Historically, the tribe fished the coast and the rivers. They ate elk and venison and hunted small game. Forests provided materials for their clothes. Increasing population to the area confined these traditional ways of food gathering. Their traditional diet was forever altered and substituted with commodities.

Chronic illness? The women promoted a Diabetes Awareness Day that included blood sugar level testing, a discussion of the disease itself, how the disease is manifested, and how to regulate activities, diet, and exercise.

What is **the** reason for the high infant mortality rate at the Cedar Bay? Perhaps there is a reason. Perhaps there are many reasons. I do not believe that they are much different from the greater society or community, but they are concentrated. Even one deviant behavior from the balanced medicine wheel can cause the whole to be unbalanced. The tribe is a microcosm. If the tribe is not healthy, we of the greater circle around the reservation, are not healthy. We are too interconnected to ignore what is happening at Cedar Bay.

The Medicine Wheel of Life is a constant rotation, a continual vigilance to stay centered. I came to the Tribe to lead a grant and to empower the women to access health care and to understand their own health behaviors. They have empowered me to speak on behalf of all. I came to share the knowledge of access to prenatal care. They taught me the medicine wheel. I came to understand their loss and grief. They helped me grieve the losses in my life. We have grieved together and celebrated together. The medicine wheel moves us in the four directions—death to birth, from ancient wisdom to the birth of new knowledge. Birth, growth and development, maturity and reflection, wisdom and death, birth and on around the wheel, again and again. It is the circle of life.

Answers

I was not meant to find an answer

Instead, to live among People

Bred with ancient wisdom

Together, we live through the seasons

And four directions

If there is an answer, let it be

To Listen

Love

Respect

Honor

Grow

Heal

Live

Each moment we are given

Spirit of the People lives among us

Their wisdom will teach us how to live

We mourn our loss and celebrate the new day

We bury our dead and give birth to a new voice

Closing Ceremony

December. The winds and storms have returned to the coast. The electricity frequently shuts off. Workers retrieve candles and emergency lights. The clinic staff waits for patients, often closing the door when no one shows. The Long House turns dark in the storm.

The administrators in Washington, who funded the work of the Women's Focus Group through the Return to Health grant will continue funding until the end of this current year. It is time to transition the work of a white public health nurse to the women of the tribal community. The final report is written. Files are reviewed. Personnel stand ready to take over the work plan. A closing ceremony is planned.

They gather: Thomas Greyhawk, Chairman of the Cedar Bay Indian Tribe; health providers from surrounding counties; members of the Health Concerns Advisory Committee which includes Dr. James Marks, Director of the Division of Reproductive Health, Centers for Disease Control in Atlanta; Dr. William Freeman, Indian Health Service from Albuquerque; Elizabeth Ward, Assistant Secretary of Health, Washington State Department of Health; Dr. Katherine Chevenaugh, The American Academy of Medicine Chicago. Caring friends from the surrounding community come. My daughter, sister, and brother-in-law all come.

Masks are displayed on tables that also hold items for potlatch. Overhead lights dim. The women begin the evening program by showing slides of their work, their trip to Washington to advocate for tribal women's health and their own stories of healing. Then, the women rise to present gifts. They honor those who contributed to the Return to Health program. They present an eagle feather to Dr. Freeman. The baby-in-the-hand tee-shirt, which has already made one cross-country trip is gifted to Dr. Marks and will now return to the east coast. Handmade beaded necklaces, dream catchers, scarves and Northwest coastal Indian mask pins are gifted to clinic staff and health providers involved with the grant program. A basket full of colorful beads is passed around. Every one selects a bead to carry home. All are honored for their presence. As the ceremony ends, Edith and Marge—the tribal health coordinator and the mental health care provider—to whom I have transitioned the program work plan, call me forward. They place a green leather medicine bag around my neck. "It contains a crystal, so that you will have clarity on your continued journey." They hand me a beautifully carved guide stick. "This will guide you on the path of the journey." They give me long and close hugs. We adjourn to the dining hall for a buffet of potluck dishes, supplemented by fresh oysters, clams, salmon and elk meat. While savoring the last of the berry cobbler, I reflect.

It has been healing for me to be in this place. It has been healthy for the community, too, as they have held gatherings, shared stories and food, danced and sang. I came from the outside to learn sensitivity to the issues of infant mortality. The tribe taught me to listen to the environment and to work with natural materials to quiet my soul. The women ask that I take the lessons I learned here and teach others. I remember the cedar trees on the island where I learned to trust and not be concerned about something over which I had no control. I visualize the forest and the trees through which I have traveled on my way to this place. I look out the window and see the ancient canoe reflected in the light of the dining hall. It carried tribal grandparents to community gatherings like this in order to commemorate and celebrate life transitions. Together, we have grieved the loss of infants, friends, parents. Together, we have honored those who have gathered by offering gifts. Supported by their friendship and knowing that the work at the Cedar Bay would continue to teach the world how to live, I mentally close the grant work and—feeling satisfied—I walk out into the stormy dark night.

Early the next morning, I gather my belongings. I place the medicine bag around my neck. I reach for the guide stick. My path, which will lead away from the tribe and back toward the city, goes through the forest. "The Grandfather will lead you," the women tell me. I close the door behind me. I start on the path that leads through the forest—where the tree is medicine.

Barbara Mould Young
December 31, 1996

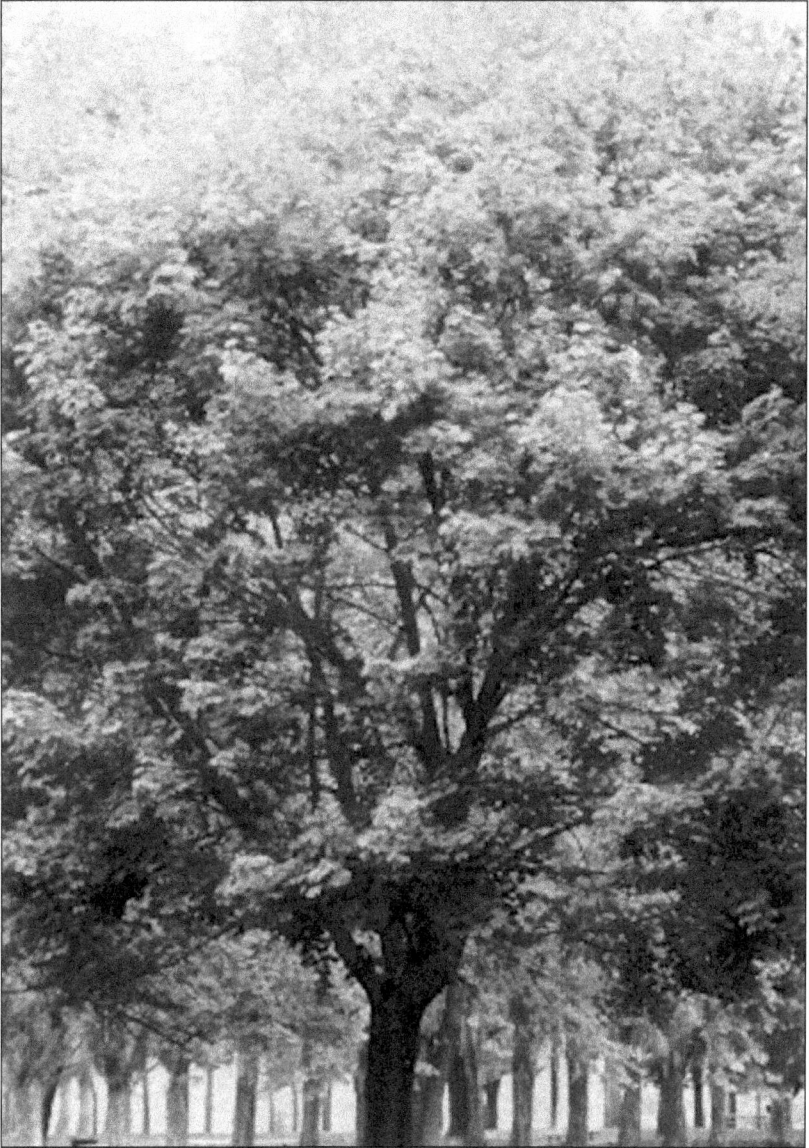

This grove of trees is part of Horse Tail State Park where Katherine and I met with the ranger to visit Tsagaglalia, the Washington State side of the Columbia River.

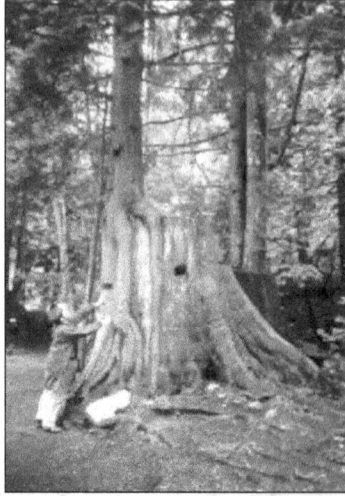

The tree stump shown with its footholds from earlier logging nourishes the next generation tree begun as a seedling on its trunk. The stump is a nurse log.

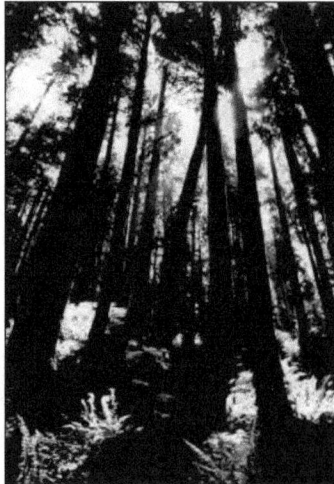

Black Elk, Sioux: "A root of the sacred tree still exists. Nurture it. Allow it to leaf. Bloom and fill with singing birds. Even in sadness and hear the singing birds. Loss in death, but re-birth. Nourish the root. The heart in the root of our human beingness."

Creation is ongoing
—Lakota

Everything has a beginning
—Kiowa

Acknowledgements

I would like to acknowledge the ancient Mound People of the Ohio Valley who taught me that life mysteries lay buried deep in the earth; co-workers and teachers in Washington state who taught me to be quiet and listen so that the lessons would reveal themselves: Mel Tonasket, Colville Federated Tribe; Louie Thadei, Aleut; Jennifer Scott, Quinault; Randy Scott, Tlingit; Ike Whitish, Hazel McKenney, Joan Shipman, Judith Altruda and Tom Anderson, Shoalwater Bay Tribe; Teresa Whitish, Tulalip and Shoalwater Bay; Bob Bajorkas, Klamath; George Anderson, Nez Perce; Midge Porter, Chinook; John Forespring, Cowlitz; Diane Moser, Cherokee, nurse practitioner who gave me a spirit bracelet for my medicine bag; Char Freeman, Blackfoot; Anna Jefferson, Lummi, who taught me to weave cedar; Trudy Marcelly, Chehalis, with whom I wove baskets; Diane, Squaxin Island, who introduced me to the sweat lodge; Dr. June Strickland, Cherokee, and Dr. Joseph Stone, Blackfoot Nation, who are professors at the University of Washington and taught me Native perspective in history, health care, and the mental health consequences of contact; Dr. Dale Croes, Cherokee, professor at South Puget Sound Community College and with whom, along with his anthropology students, I camped at the Hoko summer fishing site where the Strait of San Juan de Fuca meets the Pacific Ocean; women and girls of summer camp, South Puget Intertribal Planning Agency; Bronwyn Pughe, University of Washington Tacoma, who helped me get started and put chapters in order; Dr. Janet Primomo who provided encouragement and recommendations; Chan Mon, University of Washington Tacoma who taught me the technical skills of page and picture computer entry; Debbie Kinnaman, Lisa Sipe, Dan Adamich and Sue Folsom at Saint Martin's University who gave technical assistance; Eric Oderman and Megan Walsh, South Puget Sound Community College who gave technical assistance; Wayne McGuire, Joe Cashman, Patrick Cavendish, Marge McGinley, Paul Schaufler, and Susan Emley who read and provided comment; Elizabeth She who edited the original manuscript; Carolyn Keck who focused on copyediting; daughters Carolyn Rospierski, Katherine Flenniken and Susan YoungCrane who supported my effort to speak out concerning health care access and environmental safety; Jean Phillips and Dr. Samantha Richey who reviewed the proof; Katherine Flenniken and Charlie Keck who were the photographers; Barbara Packard, who supported publication; and Fletcher Ward who did the final editing. My thanks go to all of you.

Mosee,
Thank you,

Barbara Young
Olympia, Washington
May 2016

Resources

Baldwin, C. (1994). *Calling the Circle: The first and future culture*. Swan Raven & Co. Mill Spring, NC.

Bopp, J., Bopp, M., Brown, L. & Lane, Jr., P. (1989). *The Sacred Tree: Reflections on Native American Spirituality*. Lotus Light Publications Twin Lakes, WI.

Buhner, H. (1996). *Sacred Plant Medicine: Explorations in the practice of Indigenous herbalism*. Raven Press. Coeur d'Alene, ID.

Cajete, G. (Editor). (1999). *A People's Ecology: Explorations in sustainable living*. Clear Light Publishers. Santa Fe, NM.

Clark, E. (1953). *Indian Legends of the Pacific Northwest*. University of California Press, Berkeley, CA.

Dixon, M. & Roubideaux, Y. (2001). *Promises to Keep: Public Health Policy for American Indians & Alaska Natives in the 21st Century*. American Public Health Association. Washington, D.C.

Duran, E. & Duran, B. (1995). *Native American Postcolonial Psychology*. State University of New York. Albany, NY.

Erdoes, R. & Ortiz, A. (Editors). (1984). *American Indian Myths and Legends*. Pantheon Books, New York, NY.

Halliday, J. & Chehak, G. (1996). *Native Peoples of the Northwest: A traveler's guide to land, art, and culture*. In cooperation with the Affiliated Tribes of Northwest Indians. Sasquatch Books, Seattle, WA.

Hammerschlag, C. (1989). *The Dancing Healers: A doctor's journey of healing with Native Americans*. Harper & Row, New York. NY.

Hilbert, Vi (Taq wseblu). (1993). *Haboo: Native American Stories from Puget Sound*. University of Washington Press. Seattle, WA.

Kirk, R. & Mauzy, C. (1996). *The Enduring Forests: Northern California, Oregon, Washington, British Columbia, and Southeast Alaska*. The Mountaineers & The Mountaineers Foundation. Douglas & McIntyre, Ltd., Vancouver, B.C.

Lee, S.C. (1994). *The Circle is Sacred: A Medicine book for women*. Council Oak Books. Tulsa, OK.

National Cancer Institute. (1992). *Reducing Cancer Risks Among Native American Youth in the Northeast*. Columbia University School of Social Work. New York, NY.

Neel, D. (1995), *The Great Canoes: Reviving a Northwest Coast Tradition*. University of Washington Press, Seattle &Douglas & McIntyre, Vancouver, B.C.

Olson, W. (1991). *The Tlingit: An introduction to their culture and history*. Heritage Research. Auke Bay, Alaska.

Pavel, M. & Pavel, S. *The Teachings of du'kWXaXa'?t3w3: Sacred change for each other*. In the collection of the Seattle Art Museum. <www.coast-alsalishweaving.com>.

Roleff, T. L. (1998). *Native American Rights*. Greenhaven Press, Inc. San Diego, CA.

Schaef, A. W. (1995). *Native Wisdom for White Minds: Daily reflections inspired by the Native Peoples of the world*. One World Ballantine Books. New York. NY.

Suttles, Wayne. *Coast Salish Essays*. (1987). Talonbooks, Vancouver, B.C. & University of Washington Press, Seattle, WA.

Swan, J.G. (1857, 1966, 1977). *The Northwest Coast: or, three years' residence in Washington Territory.* Harper & Brothers, 1857; Ye Galleon Press, Fairfield, WA, 1966; Harper & Row, University of Washington Press, 1977).

Swinomish Tribal Mental Health Project. (1991). *A Gathering of Wisdoms: Tribal mental health: A cultural perspective.* Published: Office of Human Development Services and the Administration for Native Americans, Indian Health Services, Portland area, and the Washington State Division of Mental Health. Mount Vernon, WA.

Trafzer, C. E. (1990). *The Chinook.* Chelsea House Publishers, Main Line Book Co.

Wolf, E. C. (1993). *A Tidewater Place: Portrait of the Willapa ecosystem.* The Willapa Alliance. Long Beach, WA. Distributed by The Mountaineers.

Women and Girls of the Shoalwater Bay Tribal Community. (1998). *Summertime in Georgetown.* Funding for publication: Health Resources and Services Administration (HRSA), Rural Health Outreach grant.

www.ingramcontent.com/pod-product-compliance
Lightning Source LLC
Chambersburg PA
CBHW062054270326
41931CB00013B/3074